HOW TO THRIVE AS A GP TRAINEE

For my wife and children, whose patience and support made this possible – and for every GP trainee striving to grow

HOW TO THRIVE AS A GP TRAINEE

M H Shakir

MD, MRCP (UK), MRCP (London), MRCGP (UK), FRACGP (Australia)
Lead GP, Town Centre GP Surgery, Luton, UK

Scion

ISBN 9781914961816

A CIP catalogue record for this book is available from the British Library.

Scion Publishing Limited
Long Hanborough, Oxfordshire
www.scionpublishing.com

Important Note from the Publisher
The information contained within this book was obtained by Scion Publishing Limited from sources believed by us to be reliable. However, while every effort has been made to ensure its accuracy, no responsibility for loss orinjury whatsoever occasioned to any person acting or refraining from action as a result of information contained herein can be accepted by the author or publishers.

Readers should remember that medicine is a constantly evolving science and while the author and publishers have ensured that all dosages, applications and practices are based on current indications, there may be specific practices which differ between communities. You should always follow the guidelines laid down by the manufacturers of specific products and the relevant authorities in the country in which you are practising.

Although every effort has been made to ensure that all owners of copyright material have been acknowledged in this publication, we would be pleased to acknowledge in subsequent reprints or editions any omissions brought to our attention.

Typeset by Evolution Design & Digital Ltd (Kent)

Printed in the UK

Last digit is the print number: 10 9 8 7 6 5 4 3 2 1

CONTENTS

FOREWORD

Welcome to the broadest of all medical specialties. What a great book you have in your hands. Dr Shakir, a GP with a wealth of experience practising and teaching in England, has produced a worthy successor to Peter Stott's *Milestones – the diary of a trainee GP*, which I treasured during my GP training.

The life of a modern GP is, with no doubt at all, a demanding one. It draws on every part of us as human beings. It uses our every skill, and often, all our energy. I don't know how Dr Shakir managed to fit writing this book into his busy clinical life.

The book reminds trainees that they need to be kind not just to their patients, but to themselves. There is lots more wise advice, too. It will augment what trainees learn from their supervisors – and the supervisors will learn from the book too. The advice is up to date, and will remain up to date, because wisdom remains useful, even as decades and generations pass.

The British tradition of General Practice is proudly efficient and evidence-based. Dr Shakir's book is also knowledgeable; caring and humane; wise and never cynical. He has brought together top tips from the General Practice tradition and his long experience; numerous gems that will be treasured by every trainee.

Dr Jonathan Williams
BSc MSc PhD MRCGP MRCPsych

Consultant Child & Adolescent Psychiatrist,
North London Foundation NHS Trust

Honorary Associate Professor, Department of Clinical,
Education & Health Psychology, University College London

PREFACE

General practice is rarely dramatic, often unpredictable and almost always human.

When I began my journey as a GP trainee, I thought the hardest part would be mastering guidelines, learning prescribing thresholds and remembering referral pathways. With time, I realised that thriving in general practice is not about memorising algorithms. It is about learning how to sit with uncertainty, how to listen beyond words and how to make safe decisions when the picture is incomplete.

This book was born from years of clinical practice across very different settings: rural and remote communities, busy UK surgeries, out-of-hours visits, and long-term patient relationships built over decades. Each consultation, each near-miss, each difficult diagnosis and each moment of quiet reassurance has shaped the lessons within these pages.

General practice is a privilege. Patients invite us into their stories at moments of vulnerability. A frightened parent with a feverish child. A teenager asking for confidential contraception. A middle-aged man dismissing his fatigue as ageing. A woman struggling silently through perimenopause. They do not come to us with textbook presentations. They come with fear, hope, confusion and trust.

As a trainee, it can feel overwhelming. Ten minutes. Multiple problems. Uncertainty. Risk. Safeguarding. Documentation. The quiet voice in your head asking, "Have I missed something?"

You will not always have complete certainty. But you can always practise safely, thoughtfully and compassionately. That is what this book aims to support.

Within these chapters, you will find practical frameworks: what to ask, what not to miss, when to escalate and how to safety-net well. You will also find reflections. These are not shared to impress, but to illuminate. Some are stories of early detection and lives changed. Others are reminders of the weight we carry and the humility this profession demands. A few are cases that have stayed with me long after the consultation ended.

Thriving as a GP trainee is not about perfection. It is about developing judgement. It is about balancing reassurance with vigilance, curiosity with caution, empathy with efficiency. It is about learning that listening is as powerful as prescribing, and that sometimes the most important intervention is the question you almost did not ask.

General practice will stretch you. It will test your knowledge, your resilience and your emotional capacity. But it will also reward you in ways few other specialties can. You will witness continuity. You will see children grow into adults. You will support families through grief and celebrate new beginnings. You will become part of a community's fabric.

If this book does one thing, I hope it gives you confidence. Confidence to pause. Confidence to probe a little further. Confidence to trust a parent's instinct. Confidence to revisit a plan. Confidence to admit uncertainty and seek advice. Confidence to care deeply without losing yourself in the process.

Thriving is not about doing more. It is about doing what matters, consistently, safely and humanely.

This book is offered to you not as a manual of perfection, but as a companion in practice. May it steady you in uncertainty, sharpen your clinical instincts and remind you that in general practice, small decisions often shape very big outcomes.

And remember, you may not always save a life in ten minutes. But you may add ten years to it.

Hussain Shakir

ACKNOWLEDGEMENTS

No book like this is written alone. It is shaped by the people who walk alongside you throughout your professional and personal journey.

First and foremost, I would like to thank my wife, **Rehana**. More than a decade ago, she first suggested that I should write a book of this nature for GP trainees. At the time it felt like a distant idea. Over the years, her encouragement, patience and unwavering support helped turn that idea into reality. This book would not have been written without her belief in its value.

I am deeply grateful to my family, whose understanding and support allowed me the time and space to reflect on years of clinical experience and translate those lessons into writing.

My sincere thanks also go to the many colleagues, trainers, nurses, healthcare assistants and practice staff I have worked with over the years. General practice is a team endeavour. The lessons shared in this book are shaped not only by my own experiences but also by the wisdom, conversations and shared reflections of those around me.

I would also like to acknowledge the patients and communities who have trusted me with their stories. Every consultation carries a lesson. Many of the reflections in this book grew from those encounters. While identities and details have been carefully changed to preserve confidentiality, the learning they offered remains deeply appreciated.

I would like to extend my sincere thanks to **Dr Jonathan Williams**, a long-standing colleague and someone known to me through my wife's professional circle. Despite very short notice, he kindly took the time to review the manuscript in detail, offering valuable advice and thoughtful suggestions, and generously contributing a foreword. His support at a crucial stage of the book is deeply appreciated.

My special thanks go to **Dr Jonathan Ray** at Scion Publishing, who supported this project from its earliest stages and kindly accepted my original book proposal. His encouragement and thoughtful editorial input throughout the process played an important role in shaping this book. I am equally grateful to **Clare Boomer**, Production Editor at Scion Publishing, for her meticulous copy-editing, careful attention to detail and professional guidance during the production process.

Finally, this book is written for **GP trainees and early career doctors**. General practice is one of the most challenging and rewarding specialties in medicine. If the pages that follow offer reassurance, clarity or confidence at difficult moments in training, then the effort behind this book will have been worthwhile.

PART 1

STARTING OUT

"You don't have to feel ready to begin. You just have to begin – and let readiness grow with you."

CHAPTER 1
Starting out in general practice

"It's OK to feel out of your depth – every great GP once stood where you are now."

You may be reading this on your first day in a GP surgery. You've just been shown to your room – it's probably got a slightly wobbly desk, an ancient swivel chair, and a computer with more passwords than sense. You've met a multitude of colleagues: friendly receptionists, brisk nurses, and a GP trainer who speaks fast and seems brilliantly calm under pressure.

You're wearing a fresh lanyard and a cautious smile, and there's a gnawing feeling in your stomach: *What have I signed up for?*

Or maybe you're further in, perhaps six months down the line, juggling referrals, safeguarding concerns, medication queries, and trying to make your ePortfolio sound reflective and meaningful, all while thinking: *Is it meant to feel this intense?*

Either way, here's the truth: you're exactly where you need to be.

1.1 General practice isn't just another rotation

"In general practice, you don't just meet patients – you grow with them."

This isn't just another tick-box stop on the way to CCT. It's the moment medicine steps off the ward and into the front room, into schools, care homes, kitchens, and into lives.

- It's a baby with a rash whose mum is scared it might be meningitis.
- A teenage girl with anxiety, masking her fears with jokes.
- A builder with back pain who's worried it's something worse, but won't quite say it.
- A frail older woman you've seen five times this month – and deep down you know she's fading.
- Someone just diagnosed with cancer, and someone who thinks they might have it.

And it's you, in a ten-minute window, trying to listen, hold space, make safe decisions, and be kind.

It's normal to feel overwhelmed

If you feel out of your depth, you're not alone. Even the most seasoned GPs still carry some of that uncertainty. Managing risk while helping people feel safe is part of the job.

In general practice, you often won't have all the answers. What you will have is a relationship. And in this specialty, that relationship is powerful. It helps you spot the quiet cues others might miss, it helps patients trust you when things get serious. That kind of medicine is deeply human; it's about people, not just protocols, and that's why you're here.

A unique place in medicine

General practice is often misunderstood. To some, it's seen as where you 'end up' if you don't pick a hospital specialty. To others, it's the land of coughs, colds and repeat prescriptions. But to those of us who live it, it's so much more.

It's where medicine meets complexity; not just clinical complexity, but emotional, social and ethical. You'll see the same patient across chapters of their life. You'll learn their family dynamics, their fears, their resilience. And you're the one they come back to.

Continuity that matters

You'll witness things most other doctors don't.

You'll see a baby born, then attend their six-week check, then their teenage acne, and their uni-related stress. You'll help them navigate contraception, relationships, break-ups, and maybe even deliver their own child one day.

You'll support a man with Parkinson's, helping his wife through burnout, guiding them both through anticipatory grief and, one day, signing the death certificate of someone you truly knew.

This is medicine that doesn't end with discharge. It carries on. It weaves in and out of the quiet corners of people's lives.

The everyday and the extraordinary

And yes, some days will be full of routine things. You'll see hay fever, hypertension, viral illnesses, back pain. But in between will be the unspoken sadness in a teenager's silence, the domestic violence behind a *'missed pill'*, the early cancer you catch, not because it looked obvious, but because something just felt off.

You'll learn to trust your gut, to trust your patients and, slowly, to trust yourself.

> **Reflective prompts:**
> - What does 'making a difference' mean to you in general practice?
> - Can you recall a moment when you felt that?

1.2 From ST1 to ST3 – what this journey means

"You don't just become a GP by passing exams – you grow into it, one consultation at a time."

You may think of ST1 as the start of a new job. But it's more than that. It's the start of learning how to be a doctor in the community – a trusted face, a familiar voice, a calm presence when things feel uncertain.

Each year of your training shapes you differently.

ST1 – finding your feet

In ST1, everything feels new again. You've probably just come from hospital rotations, where you had structure, protocols, and a clear hierarchy. In general practice, the landscape is different. You'll have independence, and with it, a strange kind of vulnerability. There's no senior registrar sitting two beds away. It's just you in that room, with a patient, and a clock ticking towards ten minutes.

But you'll start small. And slowly, things begin to click. You'll ask for help – lots of it. You'll debrief after almost every session. You'll Google more than you're proud of. And that's all perfectly normal.

ST2 – connecting the dots

ST2 often feels like the 'middle child' of GP training. You might be rotating through hospital posts again or doing a mix of community and practice-based work. This is when things begin to make more sense.

You start recognising patterns. You see how a patient's breathlessness in A&E connects to the poorly controlled COPD you treated in clinic last month. You begin to understand the flow between services, the gaps patients fall through, and your role in catching them.

You may also sit your AKT this year – a big hurdle, but one that becomes manageable when you see it as a way to consolidate your growing experience.

You're building stamina now. Learning when to speed up, when to slow down, and how to look after yourself in the process.

ST3 – becoming the GP you're meant to be

ST3 feels like everything coming full circle. You're the senior trainee in the room. Junior colleagues ask *you* questions now. Your patients start requesting to see you again. You've learnt to make decisions with greater confidence. You've developed your style – how you explain, how you reassure, how you break bad news, how you listen.

You may be preparing for the SCA. And while it's natural to feel the pressure, it's also the time you realise how far you've come. *You are a GP,* even if your certificate hasn't arrived yet.

And beyond exams, beyond reflections and PDPs, something deeper has shifted. You start seeing yourself not just as a doctor, but as a part of your community.

> **Reflective prompts:**
> - What are you most nervous about in your GP training?
> - What support would help you navigate it better?

1.3 Why this book exists

There are plenty of GP handbooks out there: clinical guides, revision aids, exam strategy guides, evidence summaries. All of them have their place. This book isn't here to compete with them. It's here for a different reason – this book is for the moments *in between*:

- The moment you close the door after a difficult consultation and take a deep breath
- The moment you doubt yourself because you couldn't give a clear answer
- The moment you feel like you're the only one who finds this overwhelming
- The moment you realise you made a difference, even if no one said thank you.

This book is a companion for your journey. A space where you're allowed to be human. It's built from lived experience – from doctors who remember what it felt like to be new, to feel unsure, to question whether they belonged.

What you'll find here

You won't find pages and pages of protocol, but you *will* find:

- Stories and reflections from real-world practice
- Clinical confidence-builders for everyday situations
- Training tips that actually help you survive and thrive
- Wellbeing prompts, because your mental health matters too
- Kindness, tucked between every page – because this work is hard, and you deserve support.

Final thoughts – you belong here

If you've ever felt like you're not clever enough, not fast enough, not confident enough to be a GP, let this book be your reminder: *you are enough.*

The fact that you care is not a weakness. It's your strength. Keep showing up.

Keep listening. Keep learning. You're not just becoming a general practitioner. You're becoming someone's most trusted doctor. And that is a quiet kind of magic.

Reflective prompts:

- How do you look after yourself after a tough day?
- What small rituals bring you calm or grounding?

CHAPTER 2
The consultation room essentials

"It's not just what you say in the consultation – it's how you make someone feel in those ten minutes that stays with them."

This chapter offers practical, emotionally intelligent tools for navigating consultations. It balances clinical structure with human connection, acknowledging the time pressure while highlighting the opportunity for meaning, trust and healing in every ten-minute interaction.

2.1 First impressions – making people feel safe

"The consultation begins before the first question is asked."

The moment a patient walks into your room, or hears your voice on the phone, a subtle exchange begins. You may have ten minutes on the clock, but your most important work often happens in the first 30 seconds. Before you've looked at a computer, before you've thought about ICE, before you've asked a single clinical question, you've already made an impression.

And it's not about being charming or rehearsed. It's about feeling present, calm and genuinely open.

The greeting: small things, big impact

A simple smile, a warm *"Hello, come on in"*, standing up, even just briefly; these things may seem small, but they set the emotional tone.

Most patients arrive feeling slightly vulnerable, even if they don't show it. They've taken time off work, they might be worried, or they've had to build up courage just to book the consultation.

Here are a few ways to help ease that tension:

- Make eye contact as they enter (unless you're finishing something urgent on screen, in which case acknowledge that politely)
- Use their name early: *"Hi Mr Khan, lovely to meet you"*

Reflection: the first 30 seconds – when presence made the difference

It was the last consultation of an intense, back-to-back clinic. I was mentally worn down, slightly behind schedule, and still preoccupied with an unresolved safeguarding case from earlier in the day. The patient, Mrs R, was booked for 'tiredness and headaches', a familiar and seemingly non-urgent label. She was new to me.

She moved slowly, holding a notebook, frowning slightly. "Hi, please take a seat," I said, eyes on the screen. She paused before sitting, unsure. Something in that pause made me glance up. I made eye contact and offered a proper smile. That single moment changed everything.

"I wasn't sure whether to come today," she said, softly.

I nearly glossed over it. But her tone caught me – it wasn't just small talk. There was something underneath.

So I did what I should have done at the start: I pushed the laptop aside and turned fully toward her. "I'm glad you did. Tell me what's been going on."

She'd been exhausted for months, but lately she was waking in the night with panic attacks. Her husband had passed away the year before. She was trying to raise three children while quietly drowning in grief, anxiety and loneliness.

This wasn't about headaches or tiredness. It was about a woman desperately holding it all together, hoping someone might finally notice.

That consultation reminded me that sometimes, the most therapeutic moment is not the prescription or the plan – it's the space we create for people to speak their truth. All I had to do was notice her, smile and listen.

Lessons and reflections

1. **Consultations begin before the first question.**
   The tone of voice. The eye contact. The posture. These set the stage before history-taking even begins. That initial 30 seconds can open, or close, a door.
2. **Patients sense presence, or absence.**
   She nearly left without saying anything meaningful. Had I stayed in task mode, she might have asked for painkillers and gone home unheard.
3. **Connection doesn't cost time.**
   Pushing the laptop aside didn't delay my clinic. In fact, it made everything smoother. Emotional honesty often clarifies what the patient truly needs.
4. **Grief hides behind everyday labels.**
   'Headaches.' 'Tiredness.' 'Can't sleep.' Behind these lie a world of hurt we only see if we're paying attention.

- Offer a seat, even if they know the routine: *"Have a seat"* is a gentle gesture of welcome
- Tone matters – a calm, unhurried voice can do more for trust than any guideline.

Body language: your other voice

Your body language is a louder voice than you think. You communicate with far more than words. An open posture, leaning in slightly, turning your body away from the screen now and then – these actions say: *I'm here for you.*

Think about:

- facing the patient when possible
- nodding to show understanding, especially when they're opening up
- pausing before typing and letting them know why you're typing when you do: *"I'm just jotting that down so I don't miss anything important".*

It's not about being perfect, it's about being intentional.

Cultural sensitivity and neurodiversity awareness

We don't all communicate the same way. Be mindful of:

- eye contact being uncomfortable or inappropriate in some cultures
- patients with autism or anxiety who may prefer a more direct or structured interaction
- language barriers – don't rush, and use simple terms before resorting to medical jargon.

When in doubt, a little extra patience and kindness goes a long way.

Opening lines that open doors

Some common starters:

- "What's brought you in today?"
- "How can I help this morning?"
- "Tell me a bit about what's been going on."

Avoid sounding transactional. Even a small change in tone, from hurried to curious, makes all the difference.

> **Reflective prompts:**
> - Have you ever had a consultation where you felt rushed at the start?
> - How did it affect your tone? What would you do differently next time?

2.2 Structuring the ten-minute consultation

"Ten minutes isn't long, but with the right structure, it's enough to be safe, kind and clear."

One of the hardest adjustments in GP training is the time pressure; just ten minutes to greet, assess, diagnose, explain, treat and document. It can feel impossible, and some days, it is.

But structure can be your safety-net. Not a rigid script, but a rhythm – a way of moving through the consultation that helps you stay grounded, even when things get complex.

A repeatable framework

Here's a structure that many trainees (and even experienced GPs) use every day. It's not revolutionary, but it is reliable. Think of it like scaffolding: once it's second nature, you'll learn when to flex it and when to stick to it.

1. Open – let them speak

"Tell me what's been going on."

Start with an open invitation. Most patients will speak for about 60–90 seconds if uninterrupted. It's tempting to jump in, but often the clue you're looking for comes right at the end.

Show you're listening using eye contact, nods, small acknowledgements such as *"I see"* or *"Go on"*.

2. Clarify – explore ICE

Once the patient has had their say, begin to shape the conversation. This is where ICE (Ideas, Concerns, Expectations) comes in:

- **Ideas:** *"Do you have any thoughts on what it might be?"*
- **Concerns:** *"Is there anything you're particularly worried about?"*
- **Expectations:** *"What were you hoping I could do for you today?"*

It doesn't have to be formulaic, just be woven into your natural style. ICE is your shortcut to what really matters.

3. Explore – history, red flags, context

Now dig deeper and ask about:

- duration, severity and impact of symptoms
- associated symptoms
- red flags (always have a system in your head, e.g. for abdominal pain: weight loss, bleeding, fever)
- personal and social context.

You won't get it perfect every time, but that's okay. As you see more and more of the same presentations, you'll start to recognise the rhythm; the key questions will come more easily, and spotting red flags will feel like second nature.

Don't worry if it feels clunky right now; that's normal. It gets smoother.

4. Examine – when needed

If it's relevant, examine. Keep it focused, efficient and safe. Narrate what you're doing – especially with nervous or vulnerable patients.

And if you're unsure, say so. There's strength in honesty: *"I don't feel anything obvious, but I'd like to follow up."*

5. Explain – make the plan together

This is your opportunity to translate findings into meaning. Use plain language. Say what you think it is and what you're ruling out. Then check they understand:

- *"Does that explanation make sense?"*
- *"Would it help if I drew that out for you?"*

6. Plan – agree what happens next

Involve them in decision-making:

- *"We've got a couple of options and you should choose which one feels right for you."*
- *"Some people prefer to wait and watch, others want to go straight to tests. Let's talk through both."*

Be clear about prescriptions, referrals and follow-up. Write it down if needed.

7. Safety-net – protect the patient (and yourself)

Always explain what to look out for:

- *"If things get worse, or if you're not improving by next week, please come back or call us."*
- *"Here's when I'd want to hear from you again."*

And always document that clearly in your notes.

8. Close – wrap it up kindly

Before the patient leaves:

- *"Any other questions before we finish?"*
- *"Does that all make sense?"*

A good ending gives confidence and often saves return visits.

Reflective prompts:

- Have you ever missed something important because the consultation didn't feel structured?
- What might help you next time?

Reflection: the woman no one listened to – until it was nearly too late

A day etched in memory, not for its clinical complexity, but for the emotional weight it carried.

I was a GP registrar at the time, and my trainer had joined me for a consultation with a young woman presenting with chest pain and shortness of breath. As I glanced through her notes, my trainer gently remarked on her frequent attendance – more visits than there were days in a month. Her history of anxiety and depression was long-standing. His tone was subtle, but the message was clear: this wasn't a patient to be taken too seriously.

But I've never approached patients that way.

She walked in, a familiar name on the system, but a stranger to me. I introduced myself and explained my trainer's presence. With her consent, we began.

Although she had presented before with the same symptoms, I treated the consultation as if it were her first. Every patient deserves that. A history of mental illness should never cancel out the possibility of concurrent physical disease.

She was a heavy smoker, once again describing right-sided chest pain and shortness of breath. I listened, really listened, not to reassure her, but to understand. I ordered an urgent chest X-ray.

The result was devastating: a large lung mass, later confirmed as advanced lung cancer with metastases. The diagnosis had been missed before, hidden beneath the fog of assumptions and diagnostic fatigue.

She died not long after, peacefully at home. Although she had family by her side, it was my hand she held in her final moments. Her choice, not mine. I was honoured and changed.

Her story remains with me, not because I made the diagnosis, but because it reminded me what medicine is truly about: not just identifying disease, but seeing the person behind the symptoms.

Lessons and reflections

1. **Never let history cloud your judgement.**
   A patient's past – be it mental health challenges, frequent attendance or perceived behaviour – must never overshadow the need for a proper clinical assessment in the present.

2. **Every encounter deserves fresh eyes.**
   Repeat presentations may feel repetitive to us, but to the patient, they're an expression of need. Each one may still hold crucial clues.

3. **Kindness is clinical.**
   Compassion isn't an optional extra, it's a core component of care. It builds trust, encourages openness, and sometimes, offers comfort at the very end.

4. **Challenge subtle biases, even from colleagues.**
   Supervisors and peers may offer cues, consciously or not, that steer us away from curiosity and care. It's our responsibility to resist that drift. Lead quietly, by example.

2.3 Using ICE without making it robotic

"ICE isn't a script – it's a way to understand what matters to the person in front of you."

ICE is taught everywhere in GP training. It's on the curriculum, in exam prep books, and on every trainer's radar. But in practice, it can easily feel awkward, forced, or worse, irrelevant.

Done well, ICE helps you understand the real reason a patient has come in. It lets you step into their world, even briefly, and deliver care that feels personal. Done clumsily, it can sound like you're ticking boxes.

So how do you make ICE feel like a conversation, not a script?

Start with curiosity, not obligation

If you ask ICE because you're *supposed* to, patients will feel it. But if you ask because you genuinely want to understand their view, it lands completely differently.

Instead of rattling through:

- *"Do you have any ideas what your symptoms could be?"*
- *"What are your concerns?"*
- *"What were your expectations?"*

Try:

- *"Have you had any thoughts about what might be causing this?"*
- *"Is there anything in particular playing on your mind about it?"*
- *"What would a good outcome from today look like for you?"*

When to use it – and when not to

You don't need to use ICE in every single consultation, because in some, it's already obvious.

- A child with a fever? The concern is usually meningitis.
- A lump? The fear is often cancer.
- A missed period? The expectation may be pregnancy testing.

In these cases, acknowledging the likely concern out loud can be just as effective:

- *"I imagine you were worried about something serious, like meningitis?"*
- *"Did you have cancer in mind when you found the lump?"*

This still addresses the '*C*' in ICE, and shows empathy without forcing the structure.

ICE can reveal the unsaid

One of the most powerful things about ICE is what it uncovers. A patient with chest pain may really be worried it's the same thing that killed their dad. Someone with headaches may be fearing a tumour, not because the symptoms suggest one, but because anxiety is creeping in.

Don't underestimate the power of asking:

- *"What are you most worried about right now?"*

It might completely change your management, and bring them some relief.

Expectations: not always what you think

Asking what someone's hoping for doesn't mean you have to meet the expectation. It just helps manage it safely:

- *"I can see you were hoping for antibiotics, but this looks viral, so let's talk through how we can manage it well without them."*
- *"It sounds like you were hoping for a scan, but actually, based on what I've heard, we might not need to rush into that yet."*

It's about collaboration, not compliance.

> **Reflective prompts:**
> - Think of a time when asking about expectations changed your approach.
> - What did that teach you about shared decision-making?

2.4 Safety-netting – the unsung skill

"You won't always be right. That's why safety-netting exists."

In general practice, uncertainty is the rule, not the exception. You'll often see a patient at the start of their story, before the blood results, before the rash settles, before the chest pain declares itself. And in those moments, you won't always know exactly what's going on. That's okay. You're not expected to have a crystal ball.

What you *are* expected to do is think ahead. That's where safety-netting comes in. It's the skill that gently holds the space between *"wait and see"* and *"we need to act"*.

What is safety-netting, really?

It's not just a line at the end of the consultation, but it's how you:

- guide the patient through what to expect
- help them recognise when things might be going wrong
- empower them to seek help again if needed
- make it clear they won't be abandoned once they walk out the door.

When safety-netting is taken too literally

I recall a patient with suspected prostatitis who was first seen by one of my trainees. The initial assessment suggested that antibiotics were required, and he was started on a two-week course. Before leaving, he was reassured that the pain might last longer than expected, not necessarily because of ongoing infection, but due to the inflammation that can take time to settle.

A few days later, however, his condition worsened. He developed a high temperature, nausea, vomiting and increasing urinary symptoms. Instead of seeking further help, he chose to sit tight at home. In his mind, the advice about lingering inflammation explained his deterioration, so he waited rather than questioning whether something more was unfolding.

When he eventually re-presented, it was clear he had taken our words too literally. What had been intended as reassurance had unintentionally dulled his awareness of red-flag symptoms.

It was a valuable reminder to me, and to my trainee, that safety-netting advice must balance reassurance with clarity on what should prompt urgent review, and that even well-meant words can carry unintended consequences once outside the consulting room.

Don't box patients into a timeframe

A common safety-netting misstep is being too rigid with time-based advice. We've all said it: *"Come back if it's not better in a week"*.

But what if something gets worse tonight?

Patients take our words seriously, sometimes too seriously. Saying *"wait a week"* might delay care in someone who's genuinely deteriorating.

Instead, be flexible and responsive:

- *"If things deteriorate – whether that's sooner or later – please don't wait. Contact us again, call 111, or if you're really concerned, A&E or 999."*
- *"It may settle gradually, but if anything feels wrong, or just doesn't sit right, seek help."*

Be honest about what's likely

Take cough, for example. We know a post-viral cough can linger for weeks. So if we say *"come back if it lasts more than a week"*, we're setting the patient up for anxiety, and probably an unnecessary return visit. Instead, frame it realistically:

- *"These coughs often hang around for a few weeks, but if you start feeling worse, develop a temperature, or notice any new symptoms, please let us know."*

What to document

Your notes should reflect that you've considered what could go wrong and given the patient a roadmap:

- 'Safety-netting given re: possible deterioration. Advised to reconsult if worsens or new symptoms emerge. Discussed signs to monitor. No specific timeframe given.'

That's all it takes.

Tone matters

Safety-netting shouldn't frighten people. Nor should it lull them into false confidence. Aim for calm clarity:

- *"Right now, this doesn't look worrying, but it's early. If things change, just reach out."*
- *"If anything new pops up, or something doesn't feel right to you, don't hesitate to call us."*

Reflective prompts:

- Have you ever been surprised by a patient returning sooner than expected?
- What might they have needed to hear the first time?

2.5 Managing multiple problems

"You don't have to do it all today. You just have to do it well."

One of the most common trainee struggles is the *"while I'm here..."* consultation. A patient books in with a sore throat, but also wants to talk about their back pain, their repeat prescription, and a mole they're worried about.

Your heart sinks. You're only two minutes in and you can feel the list growing. So how do you manage this without rushing, resenting or letting care suffer?

Acknowledge, prioritise, plan

The first step is acknowledgement. Patients want to feel heard, even if you can't do everything today, so try:

- *"It's really helpful to know what's on your mind. Let's start with what's bothering you most."*
- *"I can see there's a few things here, shall we work through them one at a time, starting with the most urgent?"*

This makes patients feel seen and sets realistic boundaries.

Balancing patient priorities and clinical priorities

Patients often come with more than one concern. What feels most important to them may not always be the most clinically urgent.

For example, a patient may say their main priority is a facial skin lesion that bothers them cosmetically, yet in the same consultation mention chest pain with features suggesting a cardiac cause.

In these situations, your role is to acknowledge what matters to the patient, while also guiding them towards what must take priority clinically. The urgent issue should be managed immediately, with reassurance that their other concern will be given time and attention at a follow-up consultation.

This approach ensures safety while also leaving the patient feeling heard and respected.

What if it's all important?

Sometimes, everything *does* matter. You'll need to make a quick judgement call:

- Can I safely cover the essentials of all three in brief today?
- Do I need to pause and arrange a follow-up for one or two?
- Is there a pattern here – are these serial consultations for fragmented care?

And when that happens, don't be afraid to say:

- *"You've brought a few important things today, and I want to make sure each of them gets the attention it deserves. Some of these we can start on now, but to do them all safely we may need a little more time. If the issues are linked, we can extend this consultation and work through them together. If not, I can arrange for you to come back later today, either with me or another clinician, so nothing gets overlooked."*

You're allowed to protect your time and the patient's safety.

When you need to be firm

If a patient insists, or becomes upset, hold your line gently but clearly:

- *"I know it's frustrating, and I really do want to help, but I need to make sure we give each issue the time and care it deserves."*
- *"Trying to rush through everything wouldn't be safe for either of us."*

Being kind doesn't mean being overrun.

Reflective prompts:

- When you see 'multiple issues' on a patient's list, what emotions come up for you?
- How do you manage that reaction?

2.6 Ending well – leaving the door open

"A strong ending gives shape to the consultation. It tells the patient: you've been heard, and we've got a plan."

Closing the consultation well is just as important as starting it kindly. After all the listening, exploring and explaining, the final minutes are your chance to seal the plan and settle the patient. You don't need to rush, but you do need to be clear.

Wrap up with a plain summary

- *"So today we've talked about your abdominal pain, and we've agreed to..."*
- *"We've checked you over, and I'm not seeing anything serious at the moment."*

Then ask:

- *"Does that all make sense?"*
- *"Is there anything I've said today that's unclear?"*

This gives the patient a chance to ask, clarify or correct, and reminds them they're part of this, not just a passenger.

Use simple, confident language

Patients often take their cue from the way we phrase things. If we hedge unnecessarily, they may leave uncertain or anxious. Confidence in your language doesn't mean false reassurance, it means being clear, calm and straightforward.

For example, instead of saying:

- *"I think it might be okay..."*

You might say:

- *"From what I've seen today, this doesn't seem concerning, but let's keep an eye on it and review if anything changes."*

This phrase works best when paired with clear safety-netting advice. It gives reassurance without over-promising. The patient understands that, on the evidence available, there is no immediate danger, but they also know you will remain vigilant alongside them.

Clear, confident phrasing builds trust, helps patients feel safe, and avoids the uncertainty that can come from vague or overly cautious wording.

Let's ask: "is there anything else?"

The familiar *"anything else?"* question can be helpful, but it can also open the door of doom if used at the wrong moment.

Ask it too early and you risk derailing the consultation before the first concern has been explored. Ask it too late and you may find that after spending the whole consultation on one issue, the patient suddenly raises a second, more important, problem just as you're about to close.

This isn't about setting hard rules, but about knowing your patients and judging the timing. For those who frequently present with multiple issues, it can help to be clear from the outset:

Reflection: a phone call that changed more than just a result

In the bustling, multicultural town of Luton, where linguistic and cultural diversity often shape our clinical encounters in unexpected ways, I had an experience that reminded me of the deep emotional currents running beneath even the most routine interactions.

I rang a patient in his mid-forties, a heavy smoker, to discuss his recent chest X-ray. As always, I began with a calm introduction, a three-point ID check, and gently encouraged him to reflect on whether he had seen his results via the NHS app. This approach serves not only as patient education but as a gradual nudge towards shared responsibility, a step towards healthcare ownership.

Without warning, he erupted, shouting, swearing and abruptly hanging up. I sat back, stunned and momentarily hurt. The easy response, the one many clinicians would understandably default to, would have been to report the behaviour and move on. But something in me paused.

This wasn't just aggression; it was fear in disguise.

I called him back. This time, not as a GP delivering results, but as a fellow human. I apologised, genuinely acknowledging that something in my approach may have triggered his distress. I made it clear that such behaviour was not acceptable, but I also offered a compassionate lens: perhaps his anxiety about the call, about the unknown, had overwhelmed him.

That moment changed everything. He apologised, sincerely and repeatedly. He said he had never had a GP call him back after such an outburst, and that he'd been anxiously dreading the results all day.

We then proceeded with clinical clarity: antibiotics for a consolidation, a repeat chest X-ray, and, eventually, full resolution. Medically, a straightforward case. Humanly, anything but.

This story, like so many in our day-to-day work, isn't about heroism, it's about humanity. It's about remembering that, behind every outburst, there may be a story waiting to be heard.

Lessons and reflections

1. **Emotional first aid works.**
   What patients often need first is not information, but affirmation. Acknowledging their emotions without abandoning our professional boundaries can defuse even the most volatile encounters.
2. **Compassion isn't compliance.**
   Calling the patient back wasn't a concession to poor behaviour, it was a conscious, compassionate choice. One that might not be appropriate in every case, but in this one, it was transformative.
3. **No one size fits all.**
   Not every patient should be called back after aggression. Safety, context and individual judgement are paramount. But treating each case uniquely allows room for clinical courage and emotional intelligence.

4. **Clinician reflection matters.**
   Taking even a brief moment to reflect before reacting created the space for a better outcome – for the patient, and for myself.

- *"We can usually cover one concern properly in a consultation. If you've got more than one, we'll need to book another appointment so we can give each the attention it deserves."*

Used thoughtfully, this approach shows openness while protecting both safety and structure. It makes space for the patient's concerns, but also keeps the consultation manageable for you, and fair for those waiting.

- *"Have we covered what you were hoping to get out of today's appointment?"*

End with clarity and care

Final words carry weight, so end the consultation with intention:

- *"We've got a clear plan now, so do come back to us if anything changes."*
- *"Let's check in again in two weeks and see how things are going."*
- *"If you're ever unsure, please get back to us – that's what we're here for."*

Even a small gesture – such as a smile, or standing as they leave – can leave a lasting impression.

Reflective prompt:

- How might a more intentional ending change how confident the patient feels after leaving?

PART 2

CLINICAL LIFE IN GENERAL PRACTICE

"Each chapter covers a high-volume theme, focusing on the real-world presentations that dominate GP life."

CHAPTER 3

Respiratory problems

"'It's just a cough', until it isn't. Listen closely, think clearly and don't let common mean complacent."

Respiratory symptoms are a staple of general practice, especially in autumn and winter. You'll see them daily: coughs, sore throats, wheeze, breathlessness. Most will be viral, self-limiting and often fuelled by anxiety or expectation. But within the routine lie the rare and the risky: pneumonia, undiagnosed asthma, pulmonary embolism, even lung cancer.

Your role is to be vigilant, not anxious; curious, not complacent. Most are viral, but you're there to spot the one that isn't.

3.1 The presentation

A 37-year-old presents with a six-day dry cough, mild breathlessness on exertion, and a sore throat. No fever today. Smoker, but otherwise fit. Peak flow at home 'seems fine'.

This is the bread-and-butter of winter general practice; common, but layered. What seems simple could mask something more. Start broad, listen closely. You're not just treating a cough, you're managing anxiety, expectations and risk.

3.2 Key questions to ask

Don't rush past the basics. Let your curiosity lead the way.

- How long has it been going on? Is it improving or getting worse?
- Any fever, night sweats or rigor?
- What kind of breathlessness: at rest, on exertion or positional?
- Any chest pain? If so, is it sharp (pleuritic) or tight (pressure)?
- Smoking history? Baseline respiratory health?
- How is this affecting work, sleep, energy, appetite?

Reflection: the shoulder that spoke louder – a home visit that uncovered lung cancer

I was a GP registrar, carrying out what initially seemed like a routine home visit. The patient, a man in his early 80s, had been complaining of persistent left shoulder pain.

The presenting complaint suggested a straightforward musculoskeletal issue. On examination, his lungs and heart were normal, and the musculoskeletal system was unremarkable aside from some tenderness over the left shoulder, with radiation. No red flags stood out immediately. There had been no trauma, no significant joint deformity, and no acute inflammation. I could easily have opted for conservative management, offering analgesia and a plan to review.

But then, his wife quietly interjected.

She mentioned he had been losing weight recently. More strikingly, she reminded me that he was a lifelong heavy smoker. That comment nudged me to pause and reconsider. Shoulder pain in an elderly, heavy smoker deserved a second thought.

I arranged for an urgent left shoulder X-ray, just to be safe.

Later that day, radiology called the duty doctor. The X-ray had revealed a suspicious mass in the left upper lobe – an incidental finding, not what the scan was aimed at detecting.

He had shown none of the classical signs of a Pancoast tumour. There was no Horner's syndrome, no brachial plexus involvement. And yet, the pain in his shoulder turned out to be a metastatic lesion from a primary lung cancer. Further investigations confirmed advanced disease, with bony metastases to the shoulder.

He passed away peacefully just a few weeks later in a local hospice. But the family had closure. They were grateful for the timely diagnosis, for knowing what they were facing, and for being able to make the most of his remaining days.

This wasn't just about shoulder pain. It was about recognising subtle cues, respecting carer insight, and thinking holistically. We may not always change the outcome. But with curiosity and compassion, we can always impact the journey.

Lessons and reflections

1. **Never ignore context in the elderly.**
   A patient's age, smoking history and recent weight loss should prompt deeper consideration, even when the symptoms seem benign.

2. **Listen to families.**
   His wife's quiet observation prompted a critical shift in my clinical reasoning. Families often hold the missing piece of the puzzle.

3. **Shoulder pain can be more than orthopaedic.**
   Always think beyond bones and joints. Referred pain and bony metastases must stay in your differential, especially in patients with cancer risk factors.

4. **Home visits are windows into the bigger picture.**
   At home, patients and carers often open up in ways they might not in the surgery. This case reminded me how valuable those assessments can be.
5. **A timely diagnosis brings more than treatment.**
   In this case, it brought understanding, peace and preparation – elements that are just as vital as cure when time is short.

Context matters too. Ask about family members: is anyone else unwell? Any recent travel or known contact? Do they have caring responsibilities? Is this impacting their ability to function?

3.3 What you must not miss

Stay alert for red flags hiding in the ordinary:

- Pneumonia: localised chest pain, high fever, tachypnoea, focal crackles
- Life-threatening asthma: silent chest, inability to speak in full sentences, PEFR <50%
- Pulmonary embolism: sudden unexplained breathlessness, risk factors (immobility, OCP, history of DVT)
- Cancer or TB: persistent cough with haemoptysis, weight loss, night sweats.

These aren't frequent, but you're there to catch them.

3.4 The likely reality

In truth, most adult coughs are post-viral and resolve within two to three weeks. Even breathlessness can often be explained by deconditioning, inflammation or anxiety rather than infection. Sore throats? Mostly viral. Use Centor or FeverPAIN scores to guide you, but remember that they are tools, not verdicts.

Once you're confident the cough is post-viral, it helps to explain the mechanism in simple terms. This can be especially reassuring for patients during colder months:

"During a viral upper respiratory infection, the mucosal lining of the windpipe can become damaged. When that happens, it struggles to warm the air we breathe. Cold air entering the lungs can irritate or even harm them, so the body defends itself, and that defence is a cough. It's not just a leftover symptom; it's your body's way of protecting the lungs from further damage or infection. That's why the cough often worsens in autumn or winter, and especially at night, when the air is colder."

Helping patients understand this often gives them a sense of control. It validates their discomfort while guiding them through a natural recovery.

Reassurance isn't nothing, it's a clinical decision in disguise.

3.5 What to do

Viral URTI or simple cough

- Examine thoroughly: listen for signs of wheeze or focal consolidation.
- Avoid antibiotics unless the patient is systemically very unwell or at higher risk of complications (e.g. frailty, comorbidities, immunosuppression).
- Offer confident reassurance and give robust safety-netting.
- Explain the natural history: symptoms may take up to three or even four weeks to resolve.

Asthma or COPD flare

- Check peak flow and oxygen saturations if available.
- If function is clearly impaired and PEFR is significantly reduced (e.g. <75% predicted), consider prescribing a short course of oral steroids.
- Review inhaler technique, optimise regular treatment, and offer education on rescue packs if appropriate.
- Safety-net for worsening breathlessness or signs of infection.

If pneumonia is suspected

- Use CRB65 to assess severity: Confusion, Respiratory rate ≥30/min, BP ≤90mmHg systolic or ≤60mmHg diastolic, Age ≥65.
- Each CRB65 parameter scores one point, and the points are added to give the total severity score.
- If CRB65 score is 0 or 1: consider managing in primary care with oral antibiotics, clear advice and close follow-up.
- If CRB65 is 2 or more, or if clinical concern is high, arrange urgent hospital assessment.
- Document your clinical findings, decision-making and safety-netting clearly.
- Consider chest X-ray and oxygen saturations if diagnosis is uncertain or symptoms persist beyond expected timelines.

The best doctors know when not to prescribe.

3.6 Safety-netting advice

Clarity helps patients feel supported, not dismissed.

"Coughs can take two to three weeks to settle, even when it's not serious."

"If you start struggling to breathe, feel dizzy, or can't keep food down, please don't wait. Call us or 111, or visit A&E."

"If anything feels worse, get back in touch sooner."

Reflection: "it's just a virus" – when listening meant seeing more

It was a usual morning session when a 27-year-old Asian man walked in with his wife. Their visit was a follow-up, not to revisit symptoms but to question a clinical decision. They were upset that a nurse practitioner, whom he had seen days earlier for a mild respiratory illness, had not prescribed antibiotics.

His wife was particularly vocal and clearly worried. From the documented consultation, the nurse had conducted a thorough assessment. Everything pointed to a viral URTI, with no alarming signs and no red flags.

But something about this man's presence, his posture, and the concern in his wife's voice prompted me to look again.

With his consent, I re-examined him carefully. As I listened to his chest, a note of caution rose in my mind. The sounds were not quite right. They were subtle but inconsistent with a typical viral illness.

I paused and explained to them both: "Most respiratory infections do begin virally, but sometimes a secondary bacterial infection, or something more insidious, can follow."

I did not stop at reassurance. I arranged for an urgent chest X-ray the same day. The result came back later. A mass was clearly visible in his chest.

This man had never smoked in his life, yet the shadow on that film turned out to be a lung cancer, aggressive, advanced and heartbreaking.

Within three months, he passed away.

This case stays with me, not only for the tragedy of a life lost so young but also for the delicate balance we walk in primary care: between over-medicalising minor illness and missing a serious diagnosis. The difference lies in being open to changing our mind, especially when something does not sit right.

He came in over a prescription dispute, and we uncovered a terminal illness. That consultation did not save his life, but it gave him clarity, time and dignity in his final months.

Lessons and reflections

1. **Clinical notes do not tell the whole story.**
   His nurse did everything right: a thorough history, documented observations, and clear safety-netting. But illness is dynamic. What sounds viral today can evolve tomorrow.
2. **Trust your gut, and theirs.**
   His wife's concern, although rooted in frustration about antibiotics, was a signal. Family members often sense when something is not quite right. I listened to her concern rather than dismissing it as a demand.
3. **Examine again. Ask again. Reconsider.**
   A second examination, a repeat set of eyes, and a willingness to revisit an initial diagnosis can uncover life-altering pathology.
4. **Not all lung cancers are linked to smoking.**
   We must remember that young, non-smoking individuals can still harbour serious pathology. A normal demographic profile does not make someone immune to rare, devastating conditions.

Write it in your notes. Say it with care because it matters. A clear explanation is sometimes more powerful than a prescription.

3.7 Trainer's tip

There will be times you're tempted to give antibiotics *'just in case'*, to avoid complaints, or because the patient seems disappointed. Resist the urge. You're building trust not by doing what's easy, but by doing what's right and explaining why.

When patients expect antibiotics, and I explain they aren't needed, I'm often asked, "*So does that mean I don't have an infection?*". I always make it clear: "*Yes, you do have an infection but it's viral. And viral infections don't need antibiotics.*"

I explain that antibiotics are only helpful when the cause is bacterial. Taking them unnecessarily, especially during a viral illness, can actually do harm. Antibiotics disrupt the natural balance of our body's bacteria, damaging the healthy flora that live in harmony with us. They can dampen the immune response and give the virus more room to take hold.

Helping patients understand this distinction builds trust. It also strengthens their confidence in managing illness without defaulting to medication.

3.8 One-liner summary

"This sounds viral, which is uncomfortable but not dangerous right now. Let's keep an eye on it, and please let us know if anything changes, particularly if fever persists despite supportive measures, breathing worsens, or new symptoms develop."

Reflective prompts:

- Have you ever prescribed antibiotics out of uncertainty or pressure? What would you do differently now?
- What phrases do you use to explain 'just a virus' in a way that still feels respectful and reassuring?
- How do you feel when a patient challenges your decision not to prescribe?
- How do you manage that conversation?
- Think of a time when you were surprised by a respiratory diagnosis – what was missed initially, and what did it teach you?

CHAPTER 4

Cardiovascular risk and symptoms

"Prevention is quieter than intervention – but often far more powerful."

Cardiovascular issues may not be the most frequent reason patients come to the clinic, but when they do present, they are often among the most important to get right.

These are the consultations where your ability to stay calm, gather accurate information and make safe decisions can be life-saving. You do not need to be a cardiologist. You need to be a vigilant generalist, someone skilled at assessing risk, guided by clinical instinct, and confident in communicating clearly.

General practice isn't about ruling conditions in. It is about knowing what you can safely rule out.

4.1 The presentation

A 58-year-old man attends with 'a bit of chest tightness' that comes on when he walks to the shops. It settles with rest, has happened a few times, and never occurs when he is sitting still. He has a history of hypertension and smokes, but reports no nausea, collapse or sweating.

At first glance, the symptoms appear stable. However, this is exactly the kind of consultation that calls for thoughtful attention and a cautious mindset.

Chest pain is not always dramatic. That does not mean it is harmless.

4.2 Key questions to ask

To assess cardiovascular symptoms properly, your questions matter as much as your instincts. Ask clearly, listen closely, and let the story unfold before you rush to decide what it means.

- Describe the pain: is it pressure, burning or stabbing?
- When does it occur: during exertion, at rest or randomly?
- How long does it last, and what brings relief?

Reflection: The pain that didn't belong – recognising a STEMI on a surgical ward

Sometimes what looks ordinary isn't. Your eyes will often diagnose what the notes have missed.

It was 1997. I was a junior doctor on my surgical internship, having just completed six months in general medicine. The shift felt routine. Then a man in his early fifties was wheeled into the surgical ward on a stretcher. He'd been referred for epigastric pain, presumed to be a straightforward surgical case. The porter held his notes. I happened to be standing at the ward entrance as he arrived.

He was calm and speaking in full sentences, but his colour stopped me in my tracks. He looked grey and unwell – not the kind of discomfort you expect from a duodenal ulcer or biliary colic. There was no sign of active bleeding, no dramatic signs, yet something about his appearance didn't sit right.

I scanned the referral. Observations were mostly stable except for a raised heart rate. No ECG had been done. No one had asked if this pain might be cardiac rather than surgical.

At that moment, my recent medical training kicked in. I turned the stretcher around and walked him back to A&E myself. Within minutes, we had an ECG. The tracing was unmistakable: a massive anterior STEMI. The medical registrar was called, thrombolysis was started, and the patient was soon transferred to the regional cardiac unit.

He survived.

That shift became a defining memory. I learnt that being a junior doesn't mean you can't act decisively. Instinct, pattern recognition, and the courage to trust what you see – they matter more than hierarchy.

This man didn't need a surgeon. He needed a doctor who was willing to look beyond the referral letter. And that day, he got one.

Lessons and reflections

1. **Epigastric pain can be cardiac.**
   In men over 50, cardiac ischaemia may present in non-classical ways. Never exclude myocardial infarction based on location alone; always keep it in mind for upper abdominal pain.
2. **Trust your clinical instincts.**
   His observations were not alarming, but his colour was. He looked ill. That alone should always prompt action. How someone appears – their face, posture and tone – often tells you what the numbers cannot.
3. **Don't be constrained by specialty labels.**
   He was sent to surgery, but that pathway almost cost him. Diagnosis lives outside of disciplines. Your responsibility is to the patient, not the pigeonhole.
4. **Act first, justify later.**
   I could have waited. I could have accepted the referral at face value. But acting quickly saved his life. Sometimes hesitation is the greater risk.

5. **An ECG is a life-saving test.**
   It's quick, accessible and often diagnostic. If in doubt, especially with epigastric pain in an older patient, get the ECG. It might be the most important ten seconds of your day.

- Are there associated symptoms such as breathlessness, nausea, dizziness or collapse?
- Have there been previous episodes, or is there a family history of heart disease?
- What about risk factors such as smoking, diabetes, high blood pressure or raised cholesterol?

You are not just asking about symptoms. You are listening for the story behind them, the pattern that reveals the person rather than the presentation.

Sometimes the biggest decision is not what to diagnose, but whether to manage it in primary care or escalate.

4.3 What you must not miss

Always stay alert to serious underlying causes. Some of the most dangerous cardiac problems can present in quiet or misleading ways.

- Angina or acute coronary syndrome may present subtly, particularly in older patients or those with diabetes.
- Aortic dissection often causes sudden, severe chest pain that may radiate to the back.
- Pulmonary embolism can cause pleuritic chest pain, often accompanied by breathlessness.
- Arrhythmias should be suspected when there is collapse, palpitations or unexplained syncope.

These are not common presentations, but they are high-impact risks. They are the ones you do not want to miss. When your gut feeling signals caution, listen to it. You will not regret being cautious, but you might regret being casual.

4.4 The likely reality

Most chest pain seen in general practice turns out to be stable angina, musculoskeletal, or non-cardiac in origin. Common culprits include acid reflux, anxiety and chest wall strain.

- If the pain is reproducible on palpation or with movement, a musculoskeletal cause is likely.
- If the pain is vague, inconsistent, or linked to meals or emotional stress, gastrointestinal or anxiety-related causes should be considered.

Reflection: First-class diagnosis, economy-class thinking – when sub-specialty missed the systemic disease

A clean test doesn't always mean a clean bill of health. Sometimes the diagnosis is hidden in the gaps between specialties.

He was wealthy, well-connected and used to seeking only the best. In his early fifties, he began to experience a persistent discomfort in his upper abdomen. It wasn't severe, but it lingered, and he was not the kind to wait. Skipping the GP, he went straight to one of the country's leading gastrointestinal professors.

He was seen promptly, examined thoroughly, and underwent an upper GI endoscopy. The result was entirely normal. He left reassured.

A few days later, he boarded a long-haul flight to the USA. Somewhere over the Atlantic, at cruising altitude, he started to feel deeply unwell. Sweaty, weak, unsettled. He said nothing, reluctant to raise concern or cause a scene. He sat quietly, endured the discomfort, and waited for the flight to land.

When it did, he couldn't stand. Paramedics were called. He was taken off the aircraft in a wheelchair, and what followed painted a very different clinical picture:

- *He had suffered an acute ischaemic stroke*
- *He had also had a non-ST elevation myocardial infarction*
- *He was newly diagnosed with type 2 diabetes.*

His epigastric pain hadn't come from his stomach at all. It was a warning sign from his cardiovascular system. The endoscopy hadn't misfired, it had simply looked in the wrong place.

This wasn't about delayed care or limited access. It was about perspective. The specialist had done what specialists do: focus deeply on their system. But in doing so, he missed the bigger picture.

What the patient had needed was someone to ask broader questions, consider the range of differential diagnoses and examine the whole person. Not just his oesophagus, but his risk factors, his family history, his lifestyle. This was generalist work and it nearly went undone.

I still think about this man, and how close he came to catastrophe with a perfectly normal gastroscopy. It reminded me why we, as GPs, are not just gatekeepers – we are pattern recognisers. We are trained to look across systems, to ask why, and to hear what hasn't yet been said.

Lessons and reflections

1. **Epigastric pain is not always gastrointestinal.**
   In middle-aged men, especially those with risk factors, consider cardiac causes. Angina can present with epigastric discomfort, particularly in those with silent or atypical symptoms. Reflux should be a diagnosis of exclusion, not assumption.
2. **Generalists should come first.**
   While patients often seek high-profile specialists, the most useful first step is often a broad, thoughtful review from a GP or general physician. We are trained to cast wide nets and start with the system, not the symptom.

3. **Subspecialists see what they are trained to see.**
   This is not a criticism but a reality of modern medicine. A gastroenterologist will think about the stomach. A neurologist will think about the brain. The strength of generalist thinking lies in recognising overlap and asking what else this could be.
4. **Normal results don't close the case.**
   A normal OGD tells you what isn't wrong – not what is. If symptoms persist, escalate, or never quite fit, don't be falsely reassured. Reassurance should follow clinical logic, not just investigation results.
5. **Symptoms don't pause for convenience.**
   His episode on the plane could easily have been fatal. The message here is not just about systems thinking but about listening to the body, regardless of time, setting or status. Emergency symptoms can surface anywhere, even at 40,000 feet.

- Even when symptoms appear low-risk, always take the time to listen carefully, examine thoroughly, and rule out red flags before reaching a conclusion.

When you feel confident that the pain is non-cardiac, it can still be helpful to explain what cardiac pain typically feels like. A brief explanation of the difference between angina and myocardial infarction gives the patient context and confidence in your judgement. It also supports future safety.

Let them know what symptoms would warrant urgent action, when they should stop driving, and how to access emergency care if things change. A two-minute conversation like this can prevent confusion later, and can offer real peace of mind.

Record your reasoning clearly in the notes. A thoughtful explanation can support safer decision-making and reassure the patient at the same time.

4.5 What to do

If you suspect a cardiac cause, act promptly, document clearly and explain your reasoning.

If angina is suspected

- Check vital signs and assess pulse rhythm.
- Perform an ECG: ideally during symptoms, but a resting ECG can still offer helpful clues.
- Request bloods: FBC, U&Es, lipids and HbA1c.
- Consider prescribing aspirin 75mg daily, unless contraindicated (e.g. risk of bleeding, known allergy).

- Offer GTN spray if appropriate, and explain how to use it.
- Refer urgently to a Rapid Access Chest Pain Clinic (RACPC) for further assessment – this is not a cancer referral, but it should still be arranged to happen within two weeks.

If musculoskeletal pain is likely

Confirm that the pain is reproducible on palpation or movement and ensure there are no red flags.

- Document your clinical findings and your reasoning clearly.
- Offer appropriate analgesia and give advice with a plan for review.

If palpitations are the main concern

- Ask about duration, pattern, and any associated symptoms such as dizziness or blackouts.
- Perform an ECG, even if the patient is currently asymptomatic.
- Consider Holter monitoring or an event recorder if episodes are intermittent or unclear.
- Safety-net thoroughly and refer for cardiology input if any red flags are present.

The key is not to leap to conclusions but to act safely and with clarity. In chest pain presentations, it's always better to over-communicate than under-explain, both in your notes and to your patient.

4.6 Safety-netting advice

Cardiac symptoms can change course quickly. Your role is to offer clear, calm and confident advice that ensures patients know when and how to seek help. Offer safety-netting that is direct, specific and supportive:

- *"If this pain starts happening when you're resting, if it lasts longer than usual, or if it becomes more intense, please call 999 straight away."*
- *"If you collapse, feel dizzy, or find it difficult to catch your breath, seek urgent medical attention."*
- *"Don't wait until the morning; if something feels wrong, you're not wasting anyone's time, just call 111 or go to A&E for help."*

Avoid vague phrases such as 'monitor it' or 'keep an eye on it' when used in isolation. Instead, make your guidance concrete. Let patients know which symptoms are warning signs and that they can return or seek escalation without hesitation. I am not suggesting the phrase should be avoided entirely in primary care; it remains appropriate when accompanied by specific warning signs and follow-up advice.

Remember that you are not just offering information, but you are offering the patient a roadmap. The right words today could prevent a delay tomorrow.

Reflection: When 'healthy' turned harmful – the case of LoSalt and raised potassium

The answer isn't always in the blood test. Sometimes it's sitting right there on the kitchen table.

This happened in Aylesbury, during one of those quiet clinical encounters that leaves a lasting impression. A woman in her early forties, housebound but otherwise well, had routine bloods done as part of her annual review. Most of her results came back unremarkable, except for one: her potassium was raised at 5.9mmol/L.

Mild hyperkalaemia is not uncommon in general practice. It can often be attributed to sample haemolysis, ACE inhibitors or impaired kidney function. But this case didn't follow that pattern. Her renal function was normal, the sample was processed promptly, and she wasn't taking any medications known to raise potassium.

So what was going on?

I might have opted for a phone call and a second blood test, but something nudged me to visit in person. Remote reviews have their place, but they can also strip away the detail that matters. And sometimes, you need to be in the room.

She greeted me warmly. As we sat and talked, I gently explored potential causes. Had anything changed recently in her medications or diet? Any new supplements, herbal teas or lifestyle changes?

Then it came.

"I've been using LoSalt instead of table salt" *she said, quite pleased with herself.* "It's healthier, isn't it? I figured I could use a bit more of it."

There was the answer.

LoSalt is marketed as a healthier alternative to table salt. And it is, if used sparingly and with an awareness of what's inside. What many don't realise is that its main ingredient is potassium chloride. By switching to it and increasing the quantity, she had been unknowingly overloading her system with potassium.

After returning to the surgery, I checked the packaging to be sure. There it was: potassium chloride, clearly listed as the main component.

This wasn't a dramatic case. There were no hospital admissions or ECG changes. But it was a quiet success – an example of how curiosity, a home visit and a good conversation can make a genuine difference.

Lessons and reflections

1. **Ask about diet, always.**
   When bloods show a raised potassium and the usual culprits don't fit, dietary intake becomes vital. Patients often make changes with the best intentions. LoSalt, for example, is promoted as healthier, but can quietly tip potassium levels upwards.
2. **Don't assume, investigate.**
   Potassium levels above 5.5mmol/L should prompt a review. It's easy to brush off mild elevations, but doing so may delay the discovery of a preventable risk. Go through medications, renal function and diet methodically.

3. **Home visits still have their place.**
   Remote consulting is efficient, but it can flatten nuance. A visit to someone's home often reveals details you'd never uncover in a phone call. In this case, the clue was in the kitchen cupboard.
4. **Educate around over-the-counter and lifestyle products.**
   Products like LoSalt, protein powders and herbal remedies can have unintended clinical effects. Patients often don't mention them unless asked specifically. Brief education can prevent real harm.
5. **Stay curious.**
   Curiosity is a clinical asset. When the pieces don't fit, keep asking. The right question, at the right time, often unlocks the answer.

4.7 What I wish I had known

In the early stages of training, it's natural to refer more than you later might. That is not a failing – it's a safeguard.

No colleague will criticise you for being cautious when chest pain, palpitations or other potential cardiac symptoms are involved. These are high-stakes presentations, and erring on the side of safety is part of learning to become a safe and trusted generalist.

With time, you will become better at recognising patterns. You'll develop confidence in assessing which cases are low risk and can be managed within primary care. You'll also come to understand that good judgement is not just about what you know, but how willing you are to seek a second opinion when needed.

Until then, keep doing the right things: ask carefully, examine thoroughly, document clearly, and never hesitate to speak to a colleague.

4.8 One-liner summary

"Your symptoms might be related to your heart, so we'd like to get that checked properly, just to be safe."

Reflective prompts:

- When have you found yourself second-guessing a chest pain decision? What helped you resolve it?
- How do you balance caution with clarity when communicating potential heart-related concerns to patients?

CHAPTER 5

Metabolic and long-term conditions

"You might not save a life in ten minutes, but you could add ten years to it."

Managing chronic conditions may not always feel urgent, but it is some of the most transformative work you will do in general practice. These reviews are where trust is built and where patients feel seen beyond a single symptom. This is the quiet, consistent medicine that prevents strokes, heart attacks and renal failure, not through drama or high-tech intervention, but by showing up, asking the right questions and adjusting one small thing at a time. Managing long-term conditions is quiet, cumulative medicine, but it changes futures.

You do not have to be perfect. You just have to be present, informed and honest. That alone can shift the course of a person's life.

5.1 The presentation

A 62-year-old woman attends her annual diabetes review. Her HbA1c has risen from 56 to 64mmol/mol. She is on metformin and her blood pressure reads 148/90mmHg. She is unsure about starting a statin. This may feel like a routine appointment, but it is anything but routine for the patient. For her, it might feel like failure, or like she is getting worse. The way you frame this moment matters.

You are not just treating a condition. You are building a relationship over time.

5.2 Key questions to ask

Go beyond the numbers and let the conversation explore what matters to the patient.

- What is their current understanding of diabetes, cardiovascular risk and long-term outcomes?
- Are there any symptoms such as fatigue, polydipsia, urinary tract infections or vision changes?

Reflection: When TATT was Addison's – a case of intuition and timely diagnosis

He was seventeen, pale, thin and visibly worn down. He walked into my clinic with his mother, both concerned but unsure what to expect. Their complaint was one we hear often in general practice: He's tired all the time. The shorthand is familiar – TATT. Most of the time, we run the standard bloods, call back with the results and plan from there.

But something about this case felt different.

As he stepped into the room, my clinical instincts stirred. This wasn't a typical tired teenager. His complexion had a slate-grey hue. It wasn't the bronzing I had read about in textbooks, but it was off. He had lost weight. His blood pressure was low. He was tachycardic.

I had never diagnosed Addison's disease before. But I had read about it. I had seen the textbook cases, the subtle signs and the rare stories that stayed with doctors forever.

I examined him carefully and paused. Alongside the usual blood tests for TATT, I added one more: a 9 am serum cortisol.

The next afternoon, the lab called.

- *His cortisol was critically low.*
- *The suspicion for Addison's disease was confirmed.*

I called the hospital and arranged for him to be admitted that same day.

A couple of weeks later, he returned to clinic with his mother. This time, he walked in with energy and colour. He was alert. His shoulders were back. He smiled as he handed me a thank you card – simple, handwritten and heartfelt.

I have never forgotten that card. Or the boy who brought it.

It was not just about a rare diagnosis. It was a powerful reminder of why we must stay curious, stay open, and never let routine cloud our judgement. Intuition, grounded in knowledge, can change a life.

Lessons and reflections

1. **Do not let 'TATT' cloud your judgement.**
   Tired all the time is a common complaint. But occasionally, it hides something serious. Be curious, ask more, and look beyond the routine.
2. **Observation is still a superpower.**
   His colour, posture and pulse gave away more than his words. Quiet clues, spotted early, remain one of our greatest tools.
3. **Sometimes one extra test is all it takes.**
   A single 9 am serum cortisol led to a diagnosis that changed everything. Simple, accessible and easily missed.
4. **Don't wait for the classic signs.**
   Addison's disease does not always present as the textbooks say. If your gut says something's wrong, follow it.

5. **A thank you means more than you think.**
   That card sits in my drawer to this day. It reminds me of the quiet impact a GP can make – and the responsibility we hold with every consultation.

- How are they managing medication? Are there side-effects; for example, gastrointestinal upset from metformin?
- Are they maintaining their diet, physical activity and weight?
- Do they understand the relevance of blood pressure and cholesterol in the context of diabetes?

Tone is crucial, because this should feel like a conversation rather than a lecture.

5.3 What you must not miss

Chronic disease reviews are not just box-ticking exercises, but should be seen as safety reviews in disguise.

- Neuropathy: ask about tingling, burning or numb feet.
- Eyes: when was their last retinal screening?
- Cardiovascular risk: what is their QRISK score?
- Hypoglycaemia: consider the risk in older patients, particularly those on sulphonylureas.
- Adherence: are they not taking their prescribed medications but hesitant to admit it?
- Alternative therapies: are they taking any alternative treatments for their diabetes?

The numbers matter, but so does the person behind them.

5.4 The likely reality

Most patients do not 'fail' suddenly; they drift. Their HbA1c rises slowly, often with age, weight gain or life pressures. Clinic blood pressures are frequently higher than home readings. Statin hesitancy is common, not because patients are difficult, but because they are uncertain or worried.

- Do not assume they have read the patient leaflet; many have not.
- Do not rush to add medication; explore adherence and lifestyle first.
- Do not dismiss statin concerns; acknowledge, explore and explain.

A well-explained HbA1c result can do more than any leaflet ever could.

Reflection: A missed clue in the heat – diagnosing diabetes in the young

It was during a blisteringly hot summer when a 40-year-old man came in for what seemed like a routine appointment. His main concerns were excessive thirst and recent weight loss. On the surface, he appeared well and his observations were unremarkable. In the middle of a heatwave, it felt logical to assume he was simply dehydrated. He was advised to increase his fluid intake and monitor his symptoms. No blood tests were arranged.

A few days later, while chatting with a friend who happened to have diabetes, he was offered a quick check with a home glucometer. The reading was over 20mmol/L. Alarmed, he returned to the surgery. This time, blood tests were taken. His HbA1c came back at over 100mmol/mol, confirming a diagnosis of diabetes. Treatment was started promptly and, given his age and high glycaemic levels, he was referred to the hospital diabetes team for further assessment and support.

Fortunately, no complications had yet developed. The case stayed with me not because it was rare or dramatic, but because it was so easily missed and so easily preventable.

Lessons and reflections

1. **Classic symptoms are classic for a reason.**
   Excessive thirst and weight loss are hallmark signs of diabetes. Even during a heatwave, they deserve more than reassurance. Context can be misleading; do not let it override clinical sense.
2. **Looking well does not always mean being well.**
   Relying on clinical appearance alone is a trap. Many early or chronic conditions, including diabetes, present with minimal external signs. If symptoms do not quite fit the season or the story, look deeper.
3. **Always use the opportunity.**
   Every consultation is a chance to investigate, even briefly. A simple capillary glucose test in this case would have offered immediate clarity. Do not underestimate basic tools.
4. **Act early to avoid harm.**
   Early diagnosis of diabetes improves outcomes and helps prevent complications such as ketoacidosis and neuropathy, and hospital admissions. Delay risks escalation from manageable to critical.
5. **Patient initiative can be powerful.**
   This diagnosis was ultimately made because the patient, out of curiosity, used his friend's glucometer. Encouraging patients to stay curious, ask questions, and take ownership of their health helps close the gap when clinical judgement falters.

Reflection: When choice becomes costly – a diabetic foot catastrophe

It was April, during a family visit to a small town in Sri Lanka, when I was asked to see a woman in her early fifties. She was a mother of two and had been bed-ridden for several days. When I arrived, the problem was immediately clear. She was feverish, confused and clearly septic. Her right foot was wrapped tightly in layers of cloth, an attempt at home care applied by someone without medical experience.

As the dressings were removed, the smell of infection filled the room. Her foot was black, necrotic and beyond saving. Her diabetes had never been properly managed. She had rejected conventional treatment, relying instead on traditional medicine and well-meaning advice from neighbours. There was no clear history of injury, but the infection had spiralled fast.

This was the second case of its kind I had seen in my career. The first, many years earlier in rural Australia, had ended in a below-knee amputation. This time, the situation was even worse. She was septic and unstable. The surgical team determined that an above-knee amputation was the only chance to save her life. Despite delays in anaesthetic and the high risk involved, the operation went ahead. After surgery, her recovery was slow but steady. I later learnt that had we waited even a few hours longer, she might not have survived.

Months later, I visited her again. She greeted me in a wheelchair, smiling, alert and determined to return to work as a teacher. More importantly, she was now taking her diabetes medication regularly and engaging with her care. Still, her regret was quietly present. "If only I'd started earlier" she said, her voice steady but soft.

This case was not only about diabetes or infection. It was about trust, health beliefs and the consequences of delay. Primary care is not just about diagnosing illness; it is about recognising risk, communicating clearly and meeting people where they are, even when that involves having difficult conversations.

Lessons and reflections

1. **Delays can cost lives.**
   Diabetic foot infections are medical emergencies. Even short delays in seeking or offering treatment can mean the difference between recovery and major surgery or death.

2. **Respect beliefs, but balance them with risk.**
   Patients have the right to choose their treatment, including traditional or alternative approaches. When a choice risks serious harm, clinicians must respond clearly, with compassion and firmness.

3. **Education is an intervention.**
   Empowering patients through clear explanations about foot care, glucose control and infection risk is often more powerful than any prescription. Understanding can change behaviour.

4. **Amputation is not a failure.**
   This woman's surgery was not the end. It gave her a future. She returned to her family, her work and her life with renewed understanding and a second chance at health.

5. **Inequality is not only about access.**
   In rural or culturally distinct communities, health outcomes are shaped by trust, beliefs and habit as much as by services. Good care starts by listening, then explaining, and building trust one conversation at a time.

5.5 What to do

For rising HbA1c

- Review lifestyle: weight, physical activity and nutrition.
- Ask about missed doses, timing of medication and any side-effects.
- Consider escalation; for example, adding gliclazide or an SGLT-2 inhibitor if appropriate.
- Arrange foot checks and retinal screening if due. Repeat bloods where needed.

For raised blood pressure

- Recheck in clinic or encourage home monitoring before escalating treatment.
- Reinforce salt reduction, moderation of alcohol and weight management.
- Consider ACE inhibitors or calcium channel blockers based on age, ethnicity and comorbidities.
- Apply treatment thresholds: under 140/90mmHg for most adults and under 150/90mmHg for those over 80, unless individualised differently.

For statin conversations

- Consider starting atorvastatin 20mg, if appropriate.
- Explain clearly: *"This reduces your future risk. It doesn't mean you are unwell."*
- Monitor ALT at baseline and again at three months.

Statins do not mean you are sick, but they do help to reduce your cardiovascular risk.

5.6 Safety-netting advice

Always follow up with clarity and warmth:

- *"If you feel dizzy, lightheaded or unusually tired, please contact us."*
- *"Keep checking your blood pressure at home and let us know if it stays high."*
- *"We'll repeat your bloods soon to check how things are progressing."*

Reassure them that they are not alone between appointments.

Reflection: When a 'win' was really a warning: the case behind a falling HbA1c

He was 80, living on the rural outskirts of Lightning Ridge in New South Wales. Accompanied by his grandson, he arrived at the clinic to review his recent blood results. His tone was hopeful, his posture proud. His HbA1c had dropped significantly, from 88 to 60mmol/mol. There had been no changes in his medication and no new dietary plan, just what appeared to be a remarkable improvement.

Medicine, however, teaches us that when numbers improve without a clear reason, we should pause before we celebrate. I asked for permission to examine him and he agreed. What I found stopped me in my tracks. His skin was as pale as paper. He did not report fatigue or breathlessness, but something was clearly not right. I ordered a full blood count immediately.

The result showed a haemoglobin of 6.6g/dl, a picture of profound anaemia. The drop in HbA1c was not the result of improved glycaemic control. It was masking a chronic internal crisis. Further investigations, including a positive faecal immunochemical test (FIT) and colonoscopy, confirmed bowel cancer.

He was urgently referred, transfused, and managed by the surgical and oncology teams. Without that moment of clinical suspicion and a physical examination, the diagnosis, and his chance for timely treatment, might have been delayed. What began as a routine diabetes review became a turning point in his life and a lasting lesson in mine.

Lessons and reflections

1. **A falling HbA1c is not always good news.**
   Particularly in older adults, a significant drop in HbA1c without treatment changes should prompt concern for underlying illness, such as occult blood loss or malnutrition.
2. **Clinical examination still saves lives.**
   In the digital age, it is tempting to trust numbers alone. A simple, hands-on examination revealed what algorithms could not: severe anaemia hiding in plain sight.
3. **Anaemia can falsely lower HbA1c.**
   Changes in red cell turnover can produce deceptively low HbA1c readings. It is essential to interpret these values within the full clinical context.
4. **Routine reviews can be turning points.**
   What seemed like a standard diabetes review became a life-saving encounter. Every consultation holds hidden potential if we stay alert.
5. **Let one case change many.**
   Since this patient, I have adopted a simple rule. Any unexplained drop in HbA1c prompts me to check haemoglobin. A quick test and a quick call can sometimes be all it takes to catch a quiet crisis early.

5.7 What I wish I had known

You are not there to fix everything in ten minutes. You are there to move the dial, whether that is towards better health, improved habits or deeper understanding. You may not see the impact today, or even next month, but when one patient decides to try a statin, starts walking more, or brings their HbA1c down slightly, that is a real win.

You might not save a life in ten minutes, but you could add ten years to it.

5.8 One-liner summary

"Your numbers have changed a little. We have time and a plan to bring them back on track."

Reflective prompts:

- When did a long-term condition review last feel genuinely impactful to you? What made it so?
- How confident do you feel when explaining QRISK or discussing statins? What metaphors or examples help you connect with patients?
- What do you say when a patient hesitates about escalating medication? How do you keep the door open?
- Have you ever rushed a diabetes review and later felt something was missed? What would you do differently next time?
- What helps you remain patient and hopeful while supporting small but meaningful improvements?

CHAPTER 6

Mental health challenges

"You won't always have the answers, but showing up with empathy is already half the work."

Mental health is not a niche part of general practice, it is everywhere. It walks in disguised as fatigue, sleep issues, back pain or not feeling quite right. It may arrive quietly or unravel in tears. These are the moments where your presence matters more than your prescriptions, where your questions need to be both kind and clear, and where a patient may be opening up for the first time, not for solutions, but to feel understood.

You don't need to fix it, but you do need to hear it. Some of your most important work happens in silence.

This chapter focuses on low mood, anxiety and risk, offering a toolkit for safe, compassionate consultations.

6.1 The presentation

A 32-year-old woman tells you she has been feeling not quite right. She is tearful in the consultation, not sleeping, off sick from work and irritable at home. Her words are scattered, but what she is really saying is that she is not coping. You do not need a diagnosis in five minutes. You need to listen and open the door for honesty.

Explore gently, but do not be afraid to ask.

6.2 Key questions to ask

Think of this as emotional history-taking. Be structured, but stay human.

- When did this start, and did it come on gradually or after something specific?
- Have there been any changes in sleep, appetite, energy or interest in things they usually enjoy?

Reflection: The repeat request that raised the alarm

She was in her seventies, a patient I had not met before. Her request was simple, a repeat prescription for paracetamol for her chronic lower back pain. Routine, familiar and seemingly harmless.

A quick glance at her record made me pause. She had been issued 224 tablets of paracetamol just two weeks earlier, and the same amount two weeks before that. She was also on sertraline for depression and had a documented history of suicidal ideation. Suddenly, this was no longer routine.

I felt the weight of the prescription form differently that day. Could this be an unintentional overdose, or worse, a cry for help masked by familiarity? Paracetamol is available over the counter, but in large quantities it becomes a silent killer. I did not wait, I picked up the phone.

She answered. Calmly, she explained that her pain was constant and that she relied solely on "what the doctors prescribed". She denied using any additional over-the-counter medication. Even so, the risks were too great to ignore.

I halted further supplies and reduced future quantities to a safer level. I requested a community nurse home visit to assess for stockpiling. Although she declined a GP appointment, she agreed to attend A&E for a paracetamol level check. With her consent, I contacted the community mental health team and referred her to local wellbeing services.

Finally, I raised the case as a significant event analysis (SEA). The discussion at our practice meeting was constructive and sobering. We identified systemic vulnerabilities in repeat prescribing and developed action plans, including flagging frequent analgesic requests, mandatory reviews for patients with mental health risks and encouraging a moment of pause before approving prescriptions.

This SEA transformed a near-miss into a catalyst for safer practice. Our team walked away with a clearer understanding that vigilance does not slow us down; it protects our patients. This case reminded me that no task is truly routine. Every prescription, even for something as common as paracetamol, deserves a clinician's full attention. Most importantly, it reminded me never to lose sight of the human being behind the request.

Lessons and reflections

1. **Quantities speak loudly.**
   Large, repeated requests, particularly for high-risk medications, should never go unquestioned. Patterns in prescribing tell a story if we are willing to look.
2. **Systems support, but do not replace clinical judgement.**
   Electronic records are tools, not clinicians. It takes a human being to sense concern, notice a pattern and act on a hunch.
3. **Patient histories add meaning to data.**
   Knowing her mental health background gave essential context to the numbers, and context can save lives.

4. **Escalation is a lifeline.**
   A phone call, a home visit, a referral – these are not just administrative actions. They are moments of connection, protection and care.
5. **SEA as a culture of learning, not blame.**
   This was not about pointing fingers. It was about saying, "This could have ended differently; what will we do next time?" and using that question to build safer practice for everyone.

- Are they managing to function at work and at home?
- Have they had any thoughts of self-harm or of ending their life?
- Do they feel supported, or are they feeling alone with this?
- Is there a past history of anxiety, depression, trauma or other mental health difficulties?
- These questions might feel intrusive, but they are protective. Clarity can save lives.

Asking about suicide does not plant the idea; it can open a door to safety.

6.3 What you must not miss

Risk often hides behind vague complaints, so stay alert for:

- active suicidal thoughts, plans or intent
- a history of self-harm, particularly if it is recent or escalating
- psychotic symptoms such as hearing voices, paranoid beliefs or disordered thinking
- major functional decline; for example, not leaving the house, not eating, neglecting personal care or struggling to care for children
- domestic violence or coercive control
- undiagnosed postnatal depression, birth trauma or post-traumatic stress.

Do not assume safety, always ask.

6.4 The likely reality

Most patients will not need urgent referral. They are more likely to need:

- validation that their distress is real and understandable
- a plan, even if it is simple at first
- hope that how they feel now is not how they will always feel.

Many will benefit from guided self-help, talking therapies or lifestyle support. Medication has its place, but it is rarely a magic fix on its own.

SSRIs are not magic, but neither is doing nothing.

Reflection: The diagnosis that changed everything – recognising ADHD in a young man

For much of my medical training, neurodiverse conditions such as ADHD were barely acknowledged. They were rarely discussed, almost as if they did not exist. Until recently in the UK, ADHD was a term we hardly heard. Even many psychiatrists often labelled such patients with depression, anxiety, bipolar disorder or emotionally unstable personality disorder.

Yet ADHD has always been there throughout human history, unseen, unrecognised and untreated. Now, with increasing awareness, more clinicians are screening for ADHD, referring patients for assessment and seeing lives transformed by the right guidance, psychological support and medical treatment.

He came to see me after being released from a young offenders' institution. He was a bright teenager who had been bullied repeatedly at school. Despite his efforts to distance himself from his bullies, one day he lost his temper and lashed out. For that single assault, he was sentenced and spent time in custody.

When I met him, his frustration was palpable, but so was his potential. As he shared his story, I felt strongly that something deeper was going on. I initiated an ASRS (adult ADHD self-report scale) screening. The results were significant, so I referred him for a full ADHD assessment, which confirmed the diagnosis.

With the right support, including psychological therapy, structured guidance and medication, his life changed dramatically. Today he is thriving. No longer defined by impulsivity or frustration, he is now a high-flying banker with a bright future.

Lessons and reflections

1. **ADHD has always been there, we just did not see it.**
   For years, neurodiverse conditions such as ADHD went unrecognised. Many people were misdiagnosed with mood or personality disorders, missing the opportunity for life-changing treatment.
2. **One screen can change a life.**
   A simple ASRS questionnaire opened the door to the correct diagnosis. Sometimes the smallest step, asking the right questions at the right time, leads to the biggest change.
3. **Labels can limit or liberate.**
   Before his diagnosis, he carried labels of aggression and poor impulse control. The right label, ADHD, meant access to understanding, therapy and medication that transformed his future.
4. **Early recognition prevents lifelong consequences.**
   Untreated ADHD can contribute to disrupted education, unemployment, relationship breakdown, crime and imprisonment. Identifying and treating it early can change the trajectory of an entire life.
5. **Our role as GPs is to be curious.**
   By listening carefully, questioning patterns and using tools such as the ASRS, we can uncover conditions that others might overlook. Sometimes that quiet curiosity is what changes a patient's story.

6.5 What to do

For low mood or anxiety

- Use PHQ-9 or GAD-7 as conversational tools rather than rigid checklists.
- Signpost to trusted resources such as Every Mind Matters, Mind or local psychological therapy services (IAPT or equivalents).
- Refer to talking therapies early, even if there is a long waiting time.
- Support lifestyle changes, including sleep hygiene, regular movement, meaningful activity and reduction of alcohol or drugs.

Starting SSRIs (if appropriate)

- Start low, for example, sertraline 50mg or citalopram 20mg, in line with local guidance and the individual's profile.
- Warn about initial side-effects, such as increased anxiety, gastrointestinal upset or sleep disruption, and explain that these usually settle.
- Arrange a review in two to four weeks, or sooner if there are concerns about risk.
- Document clearly, especially around suicide risk, safety planning and informed consent.

Holding space without rushing is a skill, not a luxury.

6.6 Safety-netting advice

Language matters, so say things in a way that invites return, not retreat:

- *"If things get worse, or you feel unsafe, please get in touch. Don't wait."*
- *"There's always someone here, whether it's us, 111 or a crisis line. You're not alone in this."*
- *"You've taken a really brave step today. Let's keep that momentum going."*

6.7 What I wish I had known

You do not have to fix everything. Your empathy is already a powerful intervention. Many patients will not remember every word you said, but they will remember how you made them feel. Asking about suicide will not cause it, but not asking may leave someone alone with frightening thoughts. Lean into the discomfort. That is often where the healing starts, and where trust in you, and in help, begins to grow.

6.8 One-liner summary

"You're dealing with a lot, and you're not expected to manage it alone, so let's put some support in place."

Reflection: A tragic loss – when mental health care overlooked physical risk

She was 60, a woman burdened by profound anxiety and depression. She lived with hypertension and, like many people struggling with long-term mental illness, had difficulty staying consistent with her medications. One day, she sought help, not at her local surgery, but from a renowned professor of psychiatry in the capital.

The consultation lasted five minutes. In that time, she was started on venlafaxine at 150mg twice daily, a total of 300mg per day. There were no baseline checks, no gradual titration and no evident discussion of her physical health.

A week later, she collapsed at home. Her blood pressure on arrival by paramedics was 180/120mmHg. A CT scan showed a catastrophic intracerebral haemorrhage. Despite intensive medical care, she died four days later. She was not just a patient, she was a wife, a mother and a grandmother. Her sudden and preventable death left behind a grieving family and an urgent call for reflection.

This was not simply a rare side-effect. It was a known risk, and it was avoidable, predictable and tragic. This case is not about pointing fingers; it is about pointing forwards. It reminds us that even experienced clinicians, working in high-pressure environments, can miss crucial steps when systems do not support reflective, holistic practice.

Patients trust us to treat their whole being, not just their mind or body in isolation. That means balancing pharmacological efficacy with physiological safety. It means taking time, asking the right questions and cross-checking our assumptions. This woman did not need a powerful dose of an antidepressant that day; she needed a plan, rooted in caution, connection and clinical wisdom.

Lessons and reflections

1. **Venlafaxine is not benign.**
   At doses above 225mg, venlafaxine significantly increases blood pressure through its noradrenergic effects. For patients with existing hypertension, it should be prescribed with great caution, or sometimes not at all.
2. **Start low, go slow.**
   The golden rule in psychiatry and in medicine more broadly. For a complex patient like this, an initial dose such as 37.5mg once daily, with careful monitoring and follow-up, would have been safer and more proportionate.
3. **Baseline blood pressure checks are essential.**
   Before prescribing any medication known to elevate blood pressure, a simple reading is vital. In this case, a baseline blood pressure could have prompted re-evaluation, dose adjustment or consideration of an alternative treatment altogether.
4. **Five minutes is not enough.**
   Mental health prescribing is not a transaction, it is a clinical conversation. In five minutes, it is almost impossible to explore medical history, medication adherence, cardiovascular risk and the patient's understanding and preferences. Time is a safety tool.

5. **Medication compliance should prompt questions, not judgement.**
   Her non-compliance was not a character flaw, it was a red flag. Exploring the 'why' behind missed doses, fears or side-effects might have opened a different path and, ultimately, could have saved her life.
6. **Holistic care requires collaboration.**
   When treating patients with known comorbidities, communication with their GP or primary care team is crucial. Shared notes, flagged concerns and collaborative planning can change outcomes. A brief message or letter to her GP may have highlighted the risks and prompted a more cautious, joined-up approach.

Reflective prompts:

- How do you feel when a patient starts crying in your consultation? What is your instinctive response, and does it help them feel safe?
- Think of a time you avoided asking about suicide risk. What stopped you, and what would you do differently next time?
- What language do you use when introducing mental health medication? How do you balance honesty about side-effects with reassurance and hope?
- Have you ever felt emotionally drained after a mental health consultation? How do you decompress or reflect afterwards?
- How confident are you in managing mild to moderate mental health presentations without medication? What else would you like to learn or practise?

CHAPTER 7

Musculoskeletal pain and injury

"Most MSK pain isn't dangerous, but it still deserves your attention, empathy and clarity."

Back pain, shoulder niggles and knee stiffness are daily bread-and-butter issues in general practice. Most cases do not have red flags and do not need scans, but they all need to be taken seriously because pain affects people's lives; many patients fear the worst, worrying about slipped discs, arthritis or something serious. Your role is not just clinical, it is communicative: you are there to reassure without dismissing and to explain without overwhelming. You might say to a trainee, *"You're not just treating pain, you're treating fear, frustration and fatigue."* You might also remind them, *"Most patients aren't asking for a miracle, they're asking to be believed."*

7.1 The presentation

A 46-year-old delivery driver presents with lower back pain. He lifted particularly heavy boxes two days ago and now has stiffness in the morning that eases with movement, although it still aches by evening. There is no leg weakness and no red flags. This is a classic case of mechanical back pain, but even a classic presentation needs care.

7.2 Key questions to ask

Be systematic, but do not forget the emotional story behind the pain.

- When and how did it start?
- Does it radiate, and is there any pins and needles, numbness or weakness?
- Is it worse at night, and how long does stiffness last in the morning?
- Are there any red flags such as trauma, weight loss, fever, history of cancer or bladder and bowel changes?
- How is it impacting work, mood, sleep or mobility?
- What are they afraid it might be?

Reflection: The knee that wouldn't unlock – listening beyond 'just a sports injury'

He was 40, active and otherwise healthy. He came to see me after twisting his right knee while playing badminton. Since then, he had been experiencing pain, swelling and occasional locking of the joint. On the surface, it sounded like a typical sports injury, the sort that might settle with rest, ice and physiotherapy.

But something about his description of the 'locking' made me pause. This was more than discomfort. He described moments where his knee seemed to catch and refuse to straighten, leaving him stuck in mid-movement.

I examined him carefully. There was tenderness along the joint line and a small effusion, but what stood out most was his account of the locking episodes: sudden, unpredictable and functionally limiting. Rather than simply reassuring him and offering conservative advice, I referred him for an MRI.

The MRI revealed a bucket handle tear of the medial meniscus, a clear reason for his mechanical locking. He was promptly referred to orthopaedics and underwent arthroscopic surgery. At follow-up, his knee was stable, pain-free and fully functional again. What could have been months of frustration and worsening damage was avoided because we listened carefully and acted early.

Lessons and reflections

1. **Locking matters.**
   Mechanical symptoms such as locking, catching or giving way should always raise suspicion of structural injury, not just a 'simple sprain'.
2. **MRI is not always needed, but sometimes it is essential.**
   Many musculoskeletal injuries improve with conservative care; however, imaging can be life-changing when there are red-flag symptoms or persistent functional impairment.
3. **Active patients need active solutions.**
   For someone young, active and keen to return to sport, timely diagnosis and surgical intervention can restore not only function but also confidence and quality of life.
4. **A short consultation can change a long recovery.**
   Taking just a few extra minutes to clarify key symptoms, especially mechanical locking, can dramatically alter the course of treatment.
5. **Listen first, scan second, but do not dismiss.**
   Not every knee pain needs an MRI, but when a patient describes mechanical symptoms it is our job to listen, think carefully and act accordingly.

Ruling out serious causes is a clinical skill, not just a checklist.

7.3 What you must not miss

- **Cauda equina:** saddle anaesthesia, bladder or bowel symptoms, bilateral leg weakness.

- **Spinal fracture:** significant trauma or known osteoporosis.
- **Inflammatory back pain:** age under 45, morning stiffness lasting more than 30 minutes, night waking with pain.
- **Septic joint:** a red, swollen, hot joint with systemic features.
- **Giant cell arteritis (GCA):** particularly in patients over 50 with new shoulder pain, scalp tenderness, jaw claudication or fatigue.

Pain might not be dangerous, but it still needs managing well.

7.4 The likely reality

Most back and joint pain is mechanical. That does not make it imaginary; it makes it non-serious but still very real. Mechanical back pain often improves with movement and time. Middle-aged joint pain is frequently related to overuse, early osteoarthritis or lifestyle factors. Many patients are frightened that they have damaged something badly, even when your assessment suggests otherwise.

It's okay not to scan, because it's not always the answer.

7.5 What to do

Mechanical back pain

- Encourage movement and a return to normal routines, avoiding prolonged bed rest.
- Prescribe simple analgesia or short-term NSAIDs if appropriate.
- Avoid early imaging unless red flags are present.
- Offer or recommend physiotherapy, including self-referral where available.

Joint pain

- Examine for swelling, range of movement and warmth.
- Check inflammatory markers if indicated.
- If osteoarthritis is likely, discuss weight management, joint support and gentle exercise.
- Consider topical NSAIDs, which can be as effective as oral preparations with fewer systemic side-effects.

Overuse or tendonitis

- Give reassurance and advise rest and the use of anti-inflammatory gels or ice.
- Avoid early steroid injections unless function is significantly limited.
- Advise pacing and graded return to activity rather than complete rest.

"Good advice today can prevent a bad back from becoming a bad story."

Reflection: The inhalers that wouldn't work – seeing the whole patient

She was 68, living with COPD, and called to say her inhalers were not working. I triaged her case and arranged a face-to-face consultation, but she declined to come in and instead agreed to a telephone review with a GP. The GP reviewed her medications and adjusted her treatment as best as possible over the phone, while explaining the limitations of a remote consultation.

A couple of days later, she appeared again on the triage list, still saying her inhalers were not helping. This time, she agreed to come in.

When I reviewed her in person and looked carefully through her past medical history, I discovered something that explained everything. She had severe, burnt-out rheumatoid arthritis, with profound deformity of her hands. Her fingers were twisted and weakened, making it almost impossible for her to use her inhalers effectively. The problem was not the medication, it was her ability to use it.

With the support of our respiratory team, we arranged alternative inhaler devices that suited her needs, and referred her for a specialist inhaler technique review. Once she had a device she could manage, her symptoms improved significantly. It was a powerful reminder that sometimes the answer is not a new prescription but a new perspective, one that looks at the whole person and not just the diagnosis.

Lessons and reflections

1. **Look at the whole patient, not just the diagnosis.**
   Effective care means considering the person's overall health, abilities and past medical history, not only the presenting complaint.
2. **Telephone consultations have limitations.**
   Remote care can be efficient and convenient, but some problems can only be solved by seeing the patient in person. Physical review remains invaluable.
3. **Functional ability matters in treatment.**
   The 'best' inhaler is the one the patient can actually use. Device choice should always match the patient's physical abilities and dexterity.
4. **Past medical history is key.**
   Reviewing her history revealed the burnt-out rheumatoid arthritis that explained her struggles. Without this insight, further inhaler changes would likely have failed.
5. **Listening and looking prevent repeated consultations.**
   Taking the time to see her in person saved multiple future calls and frustrations, and gave her back some control over her COPD and her daily life.

7.6 Safety-netting advice

Clear, practical and kind safety-netting helps patients feel supported:

- *"This should gradually ease over the next few weeks. If it doesn't, or if it worsens, let us know."*
- *"If you get any numbness, leg weakness or bladder or bowel changes, please call immediately or go to A&E."*
- *"Let's touch base in a few weeks if you're not back to normal."*

7.7 What I wish I had known

You do not need to label every pain perfectly, but you do need to:

- rule out what is serious
- acknowledge the discomfort
- offer a clear plan
- arrange follow-up if needed.

It is entirely reasonable to say, *"This sounds mechanical, and that's good news"* as long as the patient leaves feeling heard rather than dismissed.

Most patients aren't asking for a miracle, but they are asking to be believed.

7.8 One-liner summary

"This sounds like mechanical pain, which is uncomfortable but not dangerous, so let's focus on movement and short-term relief."

Reflective prompts:

- When was the last time you felt pressure to arrange imaging? What did you do, and what might you try next time?
- What language do you use when explaining mechanical pain? How could you make it clearer or more reassuring?
- Think of a patient who did not seem satisfied with your MSK assessment. What might they have needed to hear or feel at that moment?
- Do you feel confident identifying red flags in back or joint pain? What resource or reminder helps anchor your approach?
- How do you balance realistic reassurance with making sure the patient feels their pain is taken seriously?

CHAPTER 8
It's never just a rash

"What looks minor can feel major, because it is on their skin, their face, their child."

Dermatology may not always feel like a core part of general practice, yet it is everywhere. Rashes, eczema, acne, bites, lumps and moles appear in your consulting room every single day. While many of these presentations are not medically urgent, they are often deeply personal. Skin conditions are visible, sometimes painful, and frequently affect children or young people. They can disrupt sleep, impact confidence, and carry emotional weight that is not immediately obvious.

Your role in these consultations rests on three key skills: calm observation, confident explanation, and a management plan that patients can realistically follow.

Because for the person sitting in front of you, it is rarely 'just a rash'. It is exhaustion from broken sleep, school days missed, social embarrassment, and self-esteem quietly eroded.

8.1 The presentation

A 9-year-old boy presents with an eczema flare following swimming. His mother is concerned that it may be infected. On examination, his knees are dry, cracked and mildly weepy. He is systemically well, afebrile and otherwise thriving.

It would be easy to treat this briskly and move on. For the parent, however, this consultation is not just about diagnosis. It is about worry, guilt, and the daily reality of creams, itching, resistance, tears and reassurance that never seems to last long enough.

Parents are not primarily looking for a label. They are looking for a plan that works tonight.

Reflection: When chest pain isn't the heart of the matter

He was 70, a quiet and gentle man, visiting family in the UK, who presented with persistent pain on the left side of his chest. The scene was instantly familiar. A worried daughter feared the worst, while the son-in-law was already reaching for his phone, keen to arrange an urgent ECG. Chest pain in an older adult carries weight, and the room filled quickly with anxiety as everyone braced themselves for a possible cardiac event.

Amid the tension and well-intentioned urgency, it was the smallest voice in the room that shifted everything. His 10-year-old granddaughter, guided perhaps by instinct or simple curiosity, gently lifted his shirt to look at his chest.

There it was. A clustered vesicular rash, clearly visible and tracking across the T4 and T5 dermatomes. Shingles. In that moment, the momentum towards cardiology stopped. No ECG was needed. No chest pain clinic referral was required. The diagnosis had been made quietly and accurately by a child who had simply decided to look.

The case was as heartwarming as it was humbling. It reminded us that not every episode of chest pain is cardiac, and not every worried family needs escalation to specialist care. Sometimes what matters most is a pause, a calm examination, and the courage to check what may seem obvious. There was also a gentle poetry to the story. That same observant granddaughter is now a junior doctor. Her clinical eye first revealed itself in her grandfather's living room, and it has only sharpened with time.

Lessons and reflections

1. **Shingles can mimic cardiac pain.**
   Left-sided chest wall pain in older adults quite rightly prompts concern about cardiac causes. However, neuropathic pain from shingles can present just as convincingly and is easily missed, particularly before the rash is fully apparent.
2. **Never skip the physical examination.**
   A simple inspection of the chest redirected the entire clinical pathway. One look saved time, eased anxiety, and prevented unnecessary investigations. Examination is not an optional extra. It sits at the very centre of safe and effective care.
3. **The power of simplicity.**
   This diagnosis did not require complex tools or advanced tests. It came from a basic clinical step, looking carefully at the area of concern. Much of good medicine still rests on simple actions performed thoughtfully and consistently.
4. **Family members can be unexpected allies.**
   Driven by concern and curiosity, this young girl demonstrated observation, attentiveness and instinct. She reminded us that good clinical thinking is not defined by age or title, but by the willingness to notice and to care.

5. **Early recognition improves outcomes.**
   Identifying shingles early allows timely antiviral treatment, reduced pain and fewer complications. It also spares patients unnecessary cardiac investigations and the distress that often accompanies them. A few extra moments of careful assessment can change the entire course of a consultation.

8.2 Key questions to ask

Avoid the temptation to simply name the rash. Understanding the story behind it will guide both your management and your reassurance.

Helpful questions include:

- Is this a flare of a known condition, or something entirely new?
- Have they noticed any triggers, such as soaps, detergents, clothing, swimming pools, pollen, pets or seasonal changes?
- Is it affecting sleep, play, concentration or school attendance?
- Are there any signs of infection, such as increasing pain, pus, swelling, spreading redness or fever?
- What treatments have they already tried, and crucially, how much and how often have they been used?

These questions help you tailor advice, avoid repeating ineffective strategies, and gently uncover misunderstandings around treatment use.

8.3 What you must not miss

Most dermatological presentations in primary care are benign. However, there are important red flags that you must recognise, so be particularly alert to:

- **Eczema herpeticum:** sudden onset of painful, clustered lesions, often with crusting and systemic symptoms such as fever.
- **Cellulitis:** particularly when involving the periorbital area or occurring over joints.
- **Drug rashes:** especially when associated with new medications, mucosal involvement or systemic features.
- **Melanoma warning signs, using the ABCDE criteria:** **A**symmetry, **B**order irregularity, **C**olour variation, **D**iameter, and **E**volution or change.

You do not need to know the name of every rash. You do need to know when to worry and when to act.

Reflection: When the rash is a sign, not the diagnosis

He was in his forties, a large man with a BMI of 38, and he came in with a problem he clearly hoped would be dealt with quickly. An itchy, uncomfortable rash in the groin. He hesitated before naming it, lowering his voice as though embarrassment were part of the diagnosis. Thrush.

He had already tried an over-the-counter antifungal cream. It helped briefly, then the rash returned. He had changed soaps, kept the area dry, worn looser clothing. Still it flared, worse with heat and long days on his feet. He wanted something stronger, something to make it go away.

In a busy surgery, it would have been easy to treat the skin and move on. Candidal intertrigo is common, particularly in skin folds, and topical treatment often works. But the recurrence gave pause. The skin was telling a story, and it felt unwise to silence it too quickly.

We talked, not in a checklist fashion, but with quiet curiosity. He mentioned tiredness that had crept in slowly. He was drinking more water than before. He was waking at night to pass urine, something he had dismissed as age and stress. His weight had increased over the years and now felt harder to shift.

The examination confirmed candidal intertrigo. Treatment mattered, but it could not be the end of the consultation. Recurrent groin thrush in a man is rarely just a local problem. It is often a clue to something systemic.

We agreed to treat the rash properly and to look wider. Blood tests were arranged, framed not as alarm but as sensible medicine. When the results came back, the picture was clear. His HbA1c was in the diabetic range. The rash had not been a minor inconvenience. It had been an early warning.

The conversation that followed was calm and practical. He was unsettled, but not shocked. We spoke about diabetes, weight, and small sustainable changes. Nothing dramatic. Just steps forward. When he returned a few weeks later, the rash was improving. He was less thirsty, sleeping better, and had started walking most evenings. Quiet progress, but real.

Once again, it reminded me how general practice works best. Not through dramatic intervention, but through noticing. By asking one extra question. By allowing a simple presentation to open a wider door.

Lessons and reflections

1. **Recurrent groin thrush in men is rarely just skin deep.**
   Repeated candidal infections should prompt consideration of underlying systemic causes rather than repeated topical treatment alone.
2. **Do not stop at the obvious.**
   Treating the rash is necessary, but understanding why it persists is where meaningful care begins.
3. **Always consider diabetes.**
   In patients with obesity, recurrent thrush is frequently an early sign of undiagnosed or poorly-controlled diabetes. A simple HbA1c can be transformative.

4. **Ask wider questions with sensitivity.**
   Groin symptoms carry embarrassment. A respectful, calm approach allows patients to share the associated symptoms that matter most.
5. **The extra step often makes the difference.**
   Good general practice lies in curiosity and context. The skin can be a window into metabolic health, if we remember to look through it.

8.4 The likely reality

In day-to-day practice, most eczema flares relate to inconsistent emollient use, under-dosing of topical steroids, or new triggers such as swimming, weather changes or unfamiliar products.

Many parents and teenagers underuse prescribed treatments due to fear of steroids or concerns about 'too many chemicals'. Most childhood rashes are viral and self-limiting.

A clear, confident explanation that a condition is common and manageable is far more reassuring than vague uncertainty.

When managing acne, remember that the clinical severity does not always reflect the emotional impact. Even so-called 'mild' acne can significantly affect confidence, social interaction, and a young person's developing identity.

8.5 What to do

Eczema flares

- Recommend generous emollient use, often at least 250g per week for children with widespread eczema.
- Prescribe an appropriate topical steroid, and use fingertip unit guidance to explain exactly how much to apply and where.
- Consider oral antibiotics only if there are clear signs of secondary bacterial infection.
- Emphasise long-term control through regular emollient use and trigger avoidance, rather than focusing solely on short-term flare treatment.

Rashes

- Assess distribution, presence of systemic symptoms, and whether the rash blanches.
- Reassure when a rash is likely viral and the child is otherwise well, while clearly explaining what warning signs to look out for.
- Be cautious about labelling a presentation as 'allergy' without a convincing history, as this can lead to unnecessary anxiety and restrictions.

Reflection: When experience is not enough

He was in his eighties, a white British man who had spent more than four decades farming in Africa before returning to the UK to spend the latter part of his life closer to family. His face told that story long before he did. Deeply sun-damaged skin, weathered and lined, the kind that comes from years of working outdoors without shade or sunscreen. He presented with a lesion on his face, something new, something he had noticed but not worried about.

The trainee who saw him first did exactly what we hope trainees will do. She looked carefully. The lesion was round but not neat, raised, non-pigmented, with irregular edges, measuring around 12mm. It did not look like a classic melanoma. There was no dark pigment, no obvious asymmetry that jumped out. But it did not feel right to her.

She brought the case to her trainer.

The trainer examined the lesion and took a different view. With years of experience behind him, he saw nothing overtly sinister. No alarming pigmentation. No bleeding. No rapid change reported. In his judgement, this could wait. It did not meet the threshold for an urgent referral. The advice was to observe and review.

The trainee accepted the guidance, but she was unsettled. Something about the lesion, and perhaps something about her own internal alarm, would not quieten. She followed the plan, but she did not let the concern go. She arranged to bring the patient back within a couple of weeks. When she saw him again, the doubt remained. This time, she trusted it. She referred him under the USC referral pathway.

The diagnosis was devastating. A rare amelanotic melanoma. By the time it was identified, it had already spread internally.

For everyone involved, it was a sobering moment. For the patient and his family, it was life-changing. For the trainee, it was painful but affirming. For the trainer, it was humbling.

This case stays with me, not because of the rarity of the diagnosis, but because of what it teaches about judgement, hierarchy, and the quiet courage it takes to trust your own clinical instincts.

Lessons and reflections

1. **Not all melanomas are pigmented.**
   Although uncommon, amelanotic melanoma exists, and does not follow textbook rules. Lack of pigment does not equal lack of risk, especially in sun-damaged skin.
2. **Sun exposure writes a long history on the skin.**
   Decades of outdoor work, especially in high UV environments, leave a cumulative burden. In older patients with significant sun damage, new lesions deserve careful and sometimes urgent consideration.
3. **Experience informs judgement, but does not replace it.**
   Senior clinicians bring pattern recognition and perspective, but experience is not infallible. Even the most seasoned eyes can miss what does not fit expectation.

4. **Trust your clinical discomfort.**
   The trainee's unease was not dramatic or absolute. It was quiet and persistent. That discomfort mattered. If your judgement tells you a referral is needed, act on it. You will not be penalised for keeping a patient safe.
5. **Training should empower, not silence.**
   Good training environments allow challenge, reflection and second thoughts. This case is a reminder that learning flows both ways, and that patient safety is best served when trainees are encouraged to think independently.

Acne

- Begin with topical treatments such as retinoids or benzoyl peroxide, and explain that irritation and dryness are common initially.
- Escalate to oral antibiotics, for example lymecycline, for moderate or widespread acne, in line with local guidance.
- Manage expectations early; improvement typically takes weeks to months, not days.
- Refer if there is scarring, significant psychological distress, or lack of response to appropriate treatment.

Skin lesions

- Use a dermatoscope if you are trained and confident.
- Take clinical photographs, with consent, for comparison over time or for peer discussion.
- Refer urgently via an urgent suspected cancer (USC) referral if criteria are met, or consider referral when patient anxiety remains high despite a reassuring assessment.

Reassurance is most effective when it is accompanied by clear advice and a practical plan.

8.6 Safety-netting advice

Good safety-netting should be specific, simple and kind. For example:

- *"If this starts spreading, becomes more painful, or your child seems unwell, please come back or contact us."*
- *"If things don't settle within one to two weeks of using the treatment exactly as we've discussed, we should review and consider next steps."*

Reassurance is strongest when patients know what to expect and when to return.

8.7 What I wish I had known

Naming a rash is not the whole job. The real value lies in explaining what it means, what to do now, and what to watch for.

Skin conditions are visible, personal and sometimes embarrassing. Patients are not looking for dermatology textbook explanations. They are looking for a clinician who takes their concern seriously, even when the condition appears clinically minor.

It is never just a rash, because it is their skin, their identity, or their child.

8.8 One-liner summary

"This looks like a flare rather than an infection, so let's calm it down and keep an eye on it. Please seek prompt medical advice if swelling spreads, fever develops, pain increases, or you feel generally unwell."

Reflective prompts:

- When was the last time you felt uncertain about a skin presentation? How did you manage that uncertainty with the patient or family?
- How do you currently explain eczema or acne management in a way that is both simple and effective?
- Have you ever under-prescribed topical steroids out of caution? What might you do differently now?
- What visual aids or language tools help you describe skin conditions confidently?
- How do you handle consultations where a patient's concern, for example, about a mole, does not align with your clinical assessment? Where do you draw the line between reassurance and referral?

CHAPTER 9
Gastrointestinal and genitourinary problems

"These are the symptoms people wait weeks to talk about, so when they do, listen properly."

Abdominal pain, changes in bowel habit and urinary symptoms are not only common in general practice, they are also inherently complex. They sit at the intersection of physical discomfort, fear of serious disease and deep embarrassment. Many patients delay raising these concerns for weeks or months. By the time they do, anxiety is often well-established, frequently driven by worries about cancer, ageing or loss of control.

Your response in these consultations needs to be calm, curious and clear. They are rarely glamorous encounters, yet they are often the ones where trust is built most firmly.

Do not allow embarrassment, yours or theirs, to delay careful thinking. This chapter focuses on lower urinary tract symptoms, bowel change, UTIs and men's health concerns, including the particular nuance required when discussing PSA testing.

9.1 The presentation

A 69-year-old man presents with increased urinary frequency, particularly nocturia, and a weaker urinary stream. There is no visible haematuria, no weight loss and no fever. He appears clinically well, yet he is clearly nervous.

This is everyday general practice, but it matters deeply to him. Beneath his measured description sits a quiet internal dialogue: is this cancer? Is this just ageing? Will I lose control of my bladder – or my independence?

In this context, a PSA test is not a simple tick-box investigation, it is the beginning of a conversation.

Reflection: From grief to gratitude – a transplant that transformed a life

It began in the outback, in a remote part of New South Wales. A 27-year-old man was brought to our clinic by his grandfather. He was visibly unwell: jaundiced, pale and exhausted. Only days earlier, he had buried his mother. His grief was raw and unprocessed; during the mourning period, he had been drinking heavily and admitted to 'popping paracetamol like Smarties' to manage persistent headaches and sleeplessness. Physical pain had merged with emotional distress, and self-medication had quietly escalated.

His blood tests were profoundly abnormal. His ALT was over 8000U/L, with other liver markers similarly deranged. This was not simply a red flag; it was a clinical emergency. He was in acute liver failure, most likely precipitated by paracetamol toxicity compounded by alcohol use. His condition was deteriorating rapidly.

Urgent arrangements were made for aeromedical transfer to Sydney, where he underwent liver transplantation. Against the odds, he survived.

Several months later, he returned to the clinic. He was not only physically well, but deeply changed. He had become a public health advocate, openly sharing his experience to raise awareness about the dangers of combining grief, alcohol and readily-available over-the-counter medications. His recovery was not merely clinical; it was transformational.

This was more than a case of acute liver failure. It was a collision of emotional pain, accessible harm and timely medical intervention. What began as a tragedy evolved into a story of survival, responsibility and education.

Lessons and reflections

1. **Paracetamol is not innocuous.**
   Paracetamol is widely perceived as safe because it is easily accessible. In excess, however, it can be fatal. Many patients underestimate cumulative dosing, particularly during periods of stress, grief or illness, and especially when alcohol is involved.

2. **An ALT in the thousands demands immediate escalation.**
   ALT levels in the thousands should raise immediate concern for fulminant hepatic failure. This is a medical emergency requiring urgent discussion with secondary care and rapid transfer. Delay can be catastrophic.

3. **Alcohol and paracetamol form a dangerous synergy.**
   Alcohol lowers the threshold for paracetamol toxicity and may blunt early warning symptoms. Patients experiencing emotional distress may unintentionally place themselves at significant risk by combining the two.

4. **Always ask about over-the-counter medication.**
   Non-prescription medicines are frequently under-reported. It is essential to ask explicitly about paracetamol, combination cold and flu remedies, and other over-the-counter products, particularly in patients with jaundice, abnormal liver function tests or unexplained abdominal pain.

5. **Recovery is not the end of the story.**
   Survival from life-threatening illness can be a turning point. Some patients go on to become powerful advocates for prevention and education. As clinicians, our role extends beyond treatment to supporting patients in sharing their experiences safely and constructively.

9.2 Key questions to ask

These consultations benefit from a gentle but confident exploration of symptoms. Normalising sensitive questions helps patients answer honestly and fully.

Key areas to explore include:

- How long have the symptoms been present?
- Are symptoms worse during the day or at night, how strong is the urinary stream, and is there any associated flank pain or loin discomfort?
- Is there any pain, urgency, dysuria or blood in the urine?
- Have there been any bowel changes, loss of appetite or unintentional weight loss?
- Is there a family history of prostate or bowel cancer?
- In women, are there symptoms of incontinence, prolapse, pelvic pain or recurrent infection?

Many patients will not volunteer bowel or urinary symptoms unless asked directly. Your tone often determines whether they open up or retreat into vagueness.

9.3 What you must not miss

While many gut and genitourinary presentations are benign, certain red flags require prompt recognition and action, so be alert to:

- **Urinary retention:** suprapubic discomfort, a palpable bladder, overflow incontinence.
- **Visible haematuria:** which usually warrants urgent referral.
- **New bowel change** associated with weight loss: always consider underlying malignancy.
- **Systemic features of UTI:** fever, flank or back pain, and confusion, particularly in older adults.
- **Pelvic pain with fever:** consider pelvic inflammatory disease or prostatitis.
- **Testicular swelling:** exclude torsion and testicular malignancy.

A change in bowel habit does not always indicate cancer, but it always deserves careful assessment.

Reflection: When the headache came after intimacy – listening to the pattern that matters

He was middle-aged and otherwise fit and well. His complaint was unusual, but he described it with clarity and quiet concern: severe headaches occurring exclusively during or immediately after sexual activity. These were not fleeting or mild. They were intense, throbbing pains that lasted for hours and disrupted his ability to function.

He spoke openly, without embarrassment, but with a clear sense that something was not right. His GP shared that concern. While the precise cause was uncertain, the consistency and specificity of the trigger made this very different from a routine tension headache or migraine. This was not a story to reassure away.

Neuroimaging revealed the explanation. A CT scan of the brain demonstrated multiple cerebral aneurysms. Further assessment suggested intermittent leakage during periods of raised intracranial pressure, particularly during sexual activity. The headaches were not simply painful episodes; they were warning signs.

He was referred urgently to neurosurgery, where the aneurysms were successfully coiled, significantly reducing the risk of a future subarachnoid haemorrhage. Following treatment, the headaches resolved completely, and a silent but potentially fatal threat was removed.

This diagnosis did not arise from diagnostic certainty, but from attentiveness and clinical curiosity. A GP recognised that the pattern mattered, asked the right questions, and chose investigation over assumption. In doing so, a life was very likely saved.

Lessons and reflections

1. **Patterned headaches should never be dismissed.**
   Headaches consistently triggered by specific activities – particularly sexual activity, exertion, coughing or straining – warrant careful evaluation. These presentations should prompt consideration of secondary and vascular causes rather than reflex attribution to stress or migraine.
2. **Sexual activity can unmask underlying pathology.**
   Physiological surges in blood pressure during intimacy can expose previously silent vulnerabilities such as aneurysms or other vascular abnormalities. Awareness of this link is essential and can be life-saving.
3. **Neuroimaging is justified when the story is atypical.**
   In cases of unusual, activity-related headaches, early imaging is appropriate. A CT or MRI scan can rapidly redirect care and prevent catastrophic neurological outcomes.
4. **Psychological safety enables clinical safety.**
   This patient's openness was critical to timely diagnosis. Creating a non-judgemental space where sensitive symptoms can be discussed is not a 'soft skill'; it is a core clinical competency.

5. **GPs do not need certainty, only the courage to investigate.**
   The GP did not know the diagnosis at the outset. What mattered was recognising that this presentation was not routine. Curiosity, pattern recognition and the willingness to act on unease were the true diagnostic tools.

9.4 The likely reality

In routine practice:

- LUTS in older men is most commonly due to benign prostatic hypertrophy.
- UTIs are frequent, particularly in women over 65, yet are often over-treated without adequate diagnostic certainty or culture confirmation.
- Bowel change in younger adults is frequently related to irritable bowel syndrome, stress or dietary factors, although red flags should never be dismissed.

Trust what patients tell you – and also listen for what is implied rather than stated. Pay attention to phrases such as, "*It's probably been going on longer than I first said*", which often signal minimisation driven by embarrassment or fear.

9.5 What to do

Lower urinary tract symptoms in men

- Use an IPSS to assess severity and impact on quality of life.
- Perform an abdominal examination and, where appropriate, a prostate examination.
- Exclude red flags before considering PSA testing.
- Offer PSA testing only in the absence of UTI and following a shared decision-making discussion about its benefits, limitations and potential consequences.
- Provide lifestyle advice, such as reducing evening fluid and caffeine intake, and consider an alpha-blocker such as tamsulosin if symptoms are bothersome and there are no contraindications.

Urinary tract infections

- Use dipstick testing judiciously and send urine for culture when symptoms are present, particularly in older adults, pregnant women or those with recurrent infections.
- Prescribe antibiotics in line with local guidance, taking resistance patterns into account.
- In recurrent UTIs, review hygiene practices, sexual health and contraception, and consider options such as postcoital prophylaxis or vaginal oestrogen in postmenopausal women where appropriate.

Reflection: When doing everything is not always doing the right thing

She was in her thirties and came with a concern that could not be ignored. Tiredness that had been creeping in for weeks, and now bloody diarrhoea that had persisted for two to three weeks. She was seen on the same day by a locum GP, a sensible and conscientious clinician who recognised immediately that this was not something to dismiss or delay.

The consultation was thorough. Blood tests were arranged; a faecal immunochemical test was requested; calprotectin was sent, along with stool samples for microscopy, culture and sensitivity. From a clinical safety perspective, nothing had been missed. Serious pathology had been considered, and the plan aimed to cover inflammatory bowel disease, infection and malignancy.

The patient left feeling heard. She later reflected that she was reassured by how seriously her symptoms had been taken. But reassurance did not last.

In the days that followed, something unsettled her. The number of tests. The breadth of what was being looked for. The implications, spoken and unspoken. Anxiety crept in, not only about what might be found, but about what it meant to need so many investigations at once.

At her follow-up, she raised her concerns directly, calmly and thoughtfully. She explained that she worked as a civil servant in London and was used to questioning systems and processes. She asked why so many tests had been ordered at the same time. Could they have been staggered? Was this the best use of NHS resources? Had anyone considered the psychological impact of being investigated for everything at once?

The questions caught the GP off guard. Not because they were hostile, but because they were precise and uncomfortable. The GP paused, listened, and, to her credit, reflected in real time.

She explained her reasoning. As a GP, she had wanted to be safe. She did not want to miss anything. Bloody diarrhoea in a young woman deserved attention, and she had erred on the side of thoroughness. But as the conversation unfolded, she acknowledged something important. While nothing had been unsafe, the approach may not have been proportionate.

Looking back, she felt that starting with blood tests and calprotectin to assess for inflammation and possible inflammatory bowel disease would have been reasonable. A follow-up appointment could then have been arranged to review results, symptoms and next steps. The FIT test, with its implicit link to bowel cancer, might have been better timed, introduced with context, or reserved for a later stage if indicated.

Nothing about this case was dramatic. There was no catastrophic outcome, no missed diagnosis in the traditional sense. Yet it offers a powerful lesson about modern general practice, where access to tests is broader, expectations are higher, and the line between reassurance and anxiety is thin.

The patient was not wrong to ask the questions. The GP was not wrong to want to be safe. But safety in primary care is not only about ruling out disease. It is also about sequencing, communication, and understanding how investigations land with the person sitting opposite you.

Lessons and reflections

1. **Safety includes proportionality.**
   Investigating appropriately does not always mean investigating everything at once. Thoughtful sequencing can protect patients from unnecessary anxiety while still maintaining clinical safety.
2. **Tests carry emotional weight.**
   Blood tests, stool samples and cancer screening tools are not neutral. They shape how patients understand their symptoms and their future. We must consider not only what we are testing for, but how that testing is experienced.
3. **Reasoning matters as much as action.**
   Patients may accept uncertainty more easily than unexplained thoroughness. Sharing clinical reasoning helps patients feel involved rather than overwhelmed.
4. **Be open to challenge.**
   This consultation was enriched, not undermined, by a patient who asked difficult questions. Good clinicians remain open to reflection, even when their intentions were sound.
5. **Over-investigation is not always benign.**
   While missing pathology is rightly feared, excessive investigation can also cause harm. Anxiety, misinterpretation and loss of trust can follow if testing is not carefully framed and paced.
6. **Learning does not stop at reassurance.**
   The GP had not missed anything clinically, yet still learnt something important. That is the essence of reflective practice, recognising that good care can always be refined.

Bowel change

- Ask specifically about blood in the stool, changes in consistency or frequency, tenesmus and abdominal pain.
- Consider a faecal immunochemical test (FIT) in patients over 50 with a change in bowel habit, but do not allow testing to delay referral when high-risk features are present.
- Perform an abdominal examination and, when appropriate, a rectal examination.
- Refer according to local cancer pathways if red flags are present or the FIT result is positive.

When someone finally speaks up about bowel or urinary symptoms, it is because the issue matters to them. Your listening, and your clarity, matter just as much as your investigations.

Reflection: When the test is right but the result is wrong

She was in her early forties and had been struggling for months with upper abdominal discomfort. Not dramatic pain, but a persistent gnawing sensation, worse on an empty stomach, sometimes waking her at night. She felt bloated, nauseated at times, and increasingly tired of feeling unwell without an answer. Like many patients, she had tried to manage it herself first. Antacids, dietary changes, and eventually a proton pump inhibitor prescribed elsewhere, which had helped a little but not completely.

When she came to see me, the story was familiar: epigastric pain, dyspepsia, and a sense that something was not quite right. She was worried about ulcers. She mentioned Helicobacter pylori, *having read about it herself. A stool antigen test was arranged, and she left reassured that we were finally getting closer to clarity.*

The result came back negative.

On paper, that should have been reassuring. In reality, it did not sit comfortably with the clinical picture. Her symptoms persisted. The pattern still suggested gastritis or peptic ulcer disease. She returned, confused and frustrated. If the test was negative, why did she still feel this way?

It was only then, during a careful review of the timeline, that the missing detail surfaced. She had continued taking her proton pump inhibitor right up until the stool sample was collected. No one had told her to stop. She had not thought to ask. The test had been done, but it had not been done under the right conditions.

The result was technically correct, but clinically unreliable.

We stopped the medication, explained why it mattered, and repeated the test at the appropriate interval. This time, the result was positive. The diagnosis that had felt elusive suddenly made sense. Treatment followed, and with it, genuine improvement.

What stayed with me was not the diagnosis, but the process. The test had not failed. The system around it had.

Lessons and reflections

1. **A test is only as good as the conditions under which it is done.**
   Investigations do not exist in isolation. Medications such as proton pump inhibitors can suppress *H. pylori* and lead to false negative results if not stopped in advance.
2. **Ordering a test carries responsibility.**
   Requesting an investigation is not a tick-box exercise. It includes ensuring the patient understands how to prepare, why preparation matters, and what might affect accuracy.
3. **False reassurance can delay diagnosis.**
   An unreliable negative result can be more harmful than no test at all. It may falsely close down clinical thinking and prolong patient suffering.

4. **Patients cannot follow instructions they are not given.**
Most patients want to do the right thing. Clear explanations, both verbal and written, are essential if we expect accurate results.
5. **Always return to the clinical picture.**
When results do not fit the story, pause. Revisit assumptions and ask what might be interfering. The patient's symptoms are often more truthful than the numbers on a screen.
6. **Good general practice lies in the details.**
Much of our work is not about rare diagnoses, but about getting common things right. Attention to small details can make the difference between confusion and clarity.

9.6 Safety-netting advice

Reassurance is important, but it must be paired with specific follow-up advice. Clear examples include:

- *"If you notice any blood, new pain, or changes in your appetite or energy levels, please come back to see us."*
- *"If this does not improve over the next couple of weeks, we will arrange further tests or a referral."*
- *"This is a common problem, but if anything changes, we will take it seriously."*

Concrete phrases help patients recognise when to seek help again.

9.7 What I wish I had known

These consultations are rarely quick. They involve building trust, gently unpacking fears, and occasionally delivering life-changing news. You do not need to rush, but you do need to ask clearly.

A PSA test is not a neutral act. It carries the possibility of false positives, anxiety and further invasive investigations, alongside potential benefit. Patients deserve to understand what the test can, and cannot, tell them. Sometimes, not testing immediately is the most thoughtful and clinically sound choice.

9.8 One-liner summary

"These symptoms are common and often manageable, so let's explore the cause and take this step by step."

Reflective prompts:

- How do you approach bowel or urinary symptoms when a patient appears hesitant or embarrassed? What helps you open the conversation?
- Recall a time you felt uncertain about requesting a PSA test or referring for bowel symptoms. What did you learn from the outcome?
- What is your current approach to FIT testing? When do you find it helpful, and when does it complicate decision-making?
- Have you ever missed a red flag in a gut or genitourinary consultation because it was not mentioned directly? How might you detect it next time?
- How confident do you feel explaining UTI treatment plans or recurrence risk, particularly to older adults? What is your go-to phrase?

CHAPTER 10

Women's health essentials

"Women often carry a quiet complexity in their consultations, so listen beyond the first sentence."

Women's health presentations are shaped as much by how you listen as by what you treat. Conversations about bleeding, hormones, contraception or pain often sit on years of feeling dismissed, misunderstood or too embarrassed to speak openly. A well-handled consultation can do more than address a symptom; it can restore confidence, control and dignity.

Do not wait for women to raise these issues themselves. Many have learnt, consciously or unconsciously, to suffer in silence. This chapter focuses on period problems, contraception, perimenopause and common urogenital symptoms, helping you offer clarity and choice rather than reflex prescriptions alone.

10.1 The presentation

A 44-year-old woman reports heavier and more painful periods over the past six months. She appears tired and frustrated and tells you she is "done with this." She is not using contraception. There are no red-flag features in the bleeding history. Her BMI is 28, and she is a non-smoker.

You are hearing the physical symptoms: heavier bleeding and pain. But you are also hearing something else – a deeper emotional message that she is worn down and no longer feels in control of her body.

Bleeding is often the presenting symptom. Loss of control is frequently the underlying issue.

10.2 Key questions to ask

Ask clearly, kindly and without assumptions. These consultations benefit from structure and reassurance. Key areas to explore include:

Reflection: Beyond the hormones – recognising the hidden struggles of perimenopause

She was 49 and sat opposite me with a quiet sense of unease. "I just don't feel like myself", *she said, struggling to put her experience into words. She was not tearful, nor did she meet criteria for clinical depression, but it was clear that she was not well.*

She described persistent tiredness, fragmented sleep, intermittent palpitations, and a growing irritability, particularly towards her partner and teenage children. These changes were subtle but cumulative, gradually eroding her confidence and sense of identity.

Her menstrual cycle had become unpredictable: light one month, heavy the next, occasionally absent altogether. Yet this was not her main concern. "I feel like I'm losing my spark", *she said quietly.* "My confidence has gone".

Her blood tests were unremarkable: thyroid function, iron studies, vitamin D were all within normal limits. In a time-pressured clinic, it would have been easy to attribute her symptoms to stress or low mood and move on. Instead, something prompted a single, simple question: "Could this be the perimenopause?".

Her expression shifted. No one had ever suggested it before. As we talked through the symptoms together, including disrupted sleep, mood changes, cognitive fog, emotional vulnerability and irregular periods, the pieces began to align. She cried, not from despair, but from relief. For the first time, her experience had a name.

We discussed management options, including lifestyle adjustments, nutritional support, local peer networks and hormone replacement therapy. She left with a plan, but more importantly, she left feeling seen, validated and understood.

Lessons and reflections

1. **Perimenopause is frequently the missing diagnosis.**
   Despite affecting a large proportion of women, perimenopause often goes unrecognised. Many women live with symptoms for years without anyone naming what is happening to them.
2. **The presentation is often subtle and multifaceted.**
   Perimenopause is not defined solely by hot flushes. Mood changes, sleep disturbance, cognitive difficulties, and emotional fragility may appear early and can have a profound impact on daily life and relationships.
3. **One question can change everything.**
   Asking, *"Could this be perimenopause?"* can validate years of confusion and self-doubt. That single question may be the gateway to understanding, self-compassion and effective support.
4. **Midlife pressures amplify vulnerability.**
   Women in their late forties and early fifties are often balancing demanding roles at work, at home, and in caring for others. When physiological change coincides with these pressures, the effects can be far-reaching.

5. **Normal blood tests do not exclude real suffering.**
   In perimenopause, investigations are often reassuring, yet the patient may still be struggling significantly. Listening carefully and offering a coherent explanatory framework can be as therapeutic as any medication.

- Are her cycles regular, and how heavy is the bleeding? Are there clots or flooding?
- What is the nature of the pain – cyclical or constant – and does it radiate to the back or thighs?
- What is the impact on energy levels, work, mood, sexual relationships and sleep?
- Is there any intermenstrual or postcoital bleeding?
- What method of contraception, if any, is she currently using, and does it help or worsen symptoms?
- Is her cervical screening up to date?
- Is there a family history of endometriosis, fibroids or gynaecological malignancy?

You are not simply managing hormones. You are helping someone regain a sense of normality and control.

10.3 What you must not miss

While many women's health presentations are benign, certain diagnoses must always remain on your radar. Be alert to:

- **Endometrial cancer**: any IMB, PCB or postmenopausal bleeding.
- **Anaemia**: chronic heavy periods can be profoundly depleting, both physically and emotionally.
- **Fibroids or adenomyosis**: consider when pain is severe, bleeding is heavy, or the uterus feels enlarged.
- **Sexually transmitted infections or pelvic inflammatory disease**: particularly in younger or sexually active women.
- **Ectopic pregnancy**: always consider in women of reproductive age presenting with pain or bleeding, regardless of reported contraception use.

10.4 The likely reality

Most menstrual problems have hormonal or structural explanations, yet many women have internalised them as something to endure. Heavy menstrual bleeding is common and often treatable. Hormonal contraception can be both a contributor to symptoms and an effective solution.

Reflection: Between care and confidentiality – a contraception request from a teenager

It was a quiet afternoon in a semi-rural clinic when a 15-year-old girl attended alone. Her appointment had been booked as 'period problems', but once the door closed, the real reason emerged. She wanted contraception and she was clear that she did not want her parents to know.

She was composed, articulate and notably well-informed. She had already considered her options, discounted those she did not feel suited her, and asked specifically about the combined oral contraceptive pill and the implant, referring to friends who used both. Her understanding of effectiveness, side-effects and risks was impressive. Equally striking was her fear of disclosure. "If they know" *she said quietly,* "I'll never come to the doctor again".

In a small community, where confidentiality can feel fragile, her concern was not unfounded. This consultation was no longer simply about prescribing contraception; it required careful navigation of trust, ethics and legal responsibility. I explained my duty to assess whether she could make this decision independently. We explored her relationship, screened for coercion or exploitation, discussed sexually transmitted infections and safer sex, and talked through responsibility and consequences. Her responses were thoughtful, consistent and mature.

She was Gillick competent.

I prescribed the combined oral contraceptive pill, offered follow-up, and signposted her to local sexual health services. I also explained clearly that her confidentiality would be respected unless there were concerns about her safety or wellbeing. As she stood to leave, she paused and said, "I was so scared you'd call my mum". *The relief on her face was unmistakable.*

Lessons and reflections

1. **Teenagers are often more capable than we assume.**
   Adolescents, when listened to and supported, can demonstrate a high level of insight and responsibility. Approaching these consultations without judgement allows young people to engage meaningfully in their own healthcare.
2. **Confidentiality is foundational to engagement.**
   Respecting confidentiality within legal and safeguarding boundaries creates safety and trust. Breaching it unnecessarily risks disengagement not only from contraception services, but from healthcare more broadly.
3. **Gillick competence is a clinical tool, not a barrier.**
   Gillick competence provides a structured and protective framework that supports autonomy while ensuring appropriate safeguards. In this case, it functioned exactly as intended.
4. **Our duty is to the patient before us.**
   Community expectations, parental assumptions, or personal discomfort must not override our ethical responsibility to the individual patient. Providing safe, confidential care may be pivotal to a young person's long-term health behaviours.

5. **Small consultations can have lasting impact.**
   This was not a lengthy appointment, but it was significant. Being taken seriously, spoken to honestly, and treated with respect can shape how a young person views healthcare for years to come.

Perimenopause and menopause frequently begin years before anyone names them, masked by fatigue, anxiety, low mood or irregular cycles. For many women, the experience is confusing and unsettling.

Menopause is a clinical process, but it is also an emotional transition. Your role is to acknowledge and support both.

10.5 What to do

Heavy or painful periods

- Arrange baseline blood tests such as full blood count and ferritin.
- Consider pelvic examination or transvaginal ultrasound for persistent, severe or atypical symptoms.
- Discuss treatment options including the COCP, a levonorgestrel intrauterine system (for example, Mirena), or cyclical progestogens, tailored to individual needs and risk factors.
- Recommend cycle tracking, the use of NSAIDs to reduce pain and bleeding, and simple supportive measures such as heat therapy.

Contraception

- Begin by asking what matters most to her: lighter periods, fewer hormones, reliability, flexibility or ease of use.
- Discuss LARC options, such as intrauterine devices or implants, particularly when symptom control is also a goal.
- Check blood pressure and BMI when considering the COCP and review contraindications carefully.
- Be transparent about possible side-effects, including changes in bleeding patterns, mood or skin, and encourage review if these become problematic.

Contraception is not just about preventing pregnancy. It can be a tool for symptom control, cycle regulation, and restoring confidence in one's body.

Menopause and perimenopause

- In women over the age of 45, diagnose perimenopause or menopause primarily on clinical grounds; blood tests are often unnecessary.
- Discuss HRT, including patches, gels and oral preparations, covering benefits, risks, and the primary aim of improving quality of life.

Reflection: The 'trivial' leak – when urogenital symptoms uncover deeper distress

She was 62 and greeted me with a polite smile as she sat down. "It's just a bit of leaking", *she said, almost apologetically.* "When I laugh or sneeze too hard". *She gave a small laugh herself, as if to minimise it. Her request seemed straightforward:* "Can I get something to stop it?"

Her medical records were unremarkable, with no previous documentation of urinary or vaginal symptoms. She was postmenopausal, had two prior vaginal deliveries, and no significant gynaecological or urological history. On the surface, this appeared to be a routine presentation – one we encounter frequently in general practice.

Yet something in her manner gave me pause. The self-effacing tone, the hesitation beneath the smile. I asked a few more gentle questions, and the fuller story began to emerge.

She described increasing vaginal dryness, itching and discomfort during intercourse. Intimacy had become painful and, eventually, something she avoided altogether. She had experienced recurrent urinary tract infections and had begun to limit social outings, worried about needing the toilet urgently or smelling of urine. "I used to be confident and sociable" *she said quietly.* "Now I just feel… ashamed."

Examination findings were consistent with genitourinary syndrome of menopause (GSM), including thinning of the vulvovaginal tissues, local irritation and a mild degree of prolapse. We discussed management options, including topical oestrogen, pelvic floor physiotherapy, lifestyle adjustments and relevant support services. Just as importantly, we talked about how common this is, that it was not her fault, and that effective treatments were available.

Two months later, she returned, not to complain, but to thank me; "I feel like myself again" *she said.*

Lessons and reflections

1. **Seemingly minor symptoms may conceal major impact.**
   What is presented as 'just a bit of leaking' may mask profound effects on confidence, intimacy and social participation. Listening beyond the opening line is essential.
2. **Create space for what is not easily said.**
   Many women will not volunteer symptoms such as vaginal dryness, discomfort or incontinence unless directly asked. A few sensitive questions from us may unlock months or years of silent distress.
3. **Recognise genitourinary syndrome of menopause.**
   GSM is common yet frequently under-diagnosed. Management is not only hormonal; it involves validation, explanation, and restoring comfort and dignity in daily life and relationships.

4. **Holistic general practice makes a tangible difference.**
   This consultation was not simply about prescribing or containment products. It required listening, examination, explanation and follow-up. General practice is uniquely placed to offer this continuity and breadth of care.
5. **Acknowledgement is empowering.**
   For many women, hearing 'this is common and treatable' is transformative. It reframes shame into action and restores a sense of control over their own bodies.

- Offer vaginal oestrogen for urogenital symptoms such as dryness, discomfort or recurrent UTIs. This is usually safe, even in some women with a history of breast cancer, when guided by specialist advice and current guidelines.
- Support lifestyle measures including weight-bearing exercise, balanced nutrition, alcohol moderation, smoking cessation, and psychological support for mood and sleep disturbance.

10.6 Safety-netting advice

Effective safety-netting should be clear, practical and reassuring. Examples include:

- *"If your bleeding changes suddenly, becomes much heavier, lasts longer, or becomes unpredictable, please come back so we can review this."*
- *"If you notice bleeding after sex or between periods, please book an appointment promptly so we can assess it carefully."*
- *"We can try this approach for a few months. If it does not help enough, we can review and look at other options together."*

10.7 What I wish I had known

There is real power in a well-framed question such as, "*What would feeling in control look like for you?*" Many women respond with, "*I thought this was normal*", a sentence that often carries years of minimised distress and unspoken frustration.

Common symptoms are not necessarily acceptable symptoms. Seeing similar problems frequently should never lead to minimising their impact.

Earlier in my practice, I did not always hear what was not being said. Now, I try to listen as carefully for the pauses, hesitations and quiet admissions of "*I've just put up with it*" as for the spoken words.

Reflection: A hidden cut – the case that spoke without words

This case was shared at one of our monthly clinical meetings by an experienced practice nurse. It involved a 23-year-old woman attending for her first cervical smear. British-born, with family origins in East Africa, she had recently registered with the practice and this was her first sustained contact with primary care as an adult.

She was quiet, polite and composed throughout the consultation. The appointment had been booked as a routine cervical screening. There were no reported symptoms and no expressed concerns – a seemingly straightforward check-up.

During the examination, the nurse paused. The external genital anatomy was altered. Scar tissue had replaced normal labial structures. The clitoris was not visible, and the vaginal opening was significantly narrowed. It became clear that this young woman had undergone Type III female genital mutilation (FGM), also known as infibulation.

She had not mentioned it. No one had previously asked.

The nurse stopped the examination gently and spoke with calm compassion, checking in with her before proceeding further. The patient responded quietly, "Yes. It happened when I was little. I don't really talk about it".

They discussed her right to appropriate care and her right to safety. The nurse explained that specialist support was available and outlined referral to the local FGM clinic, including physical and psychological care. The patient agreed. As she was leaving, she said, "You're the first person who's ever asked me about this".

Lessons and reflections

1. **FGM is a UK safeguarding issue, not a distant problem.**
   FGM affects thousands of women living in the UK. Many were subjected to it as children, often overseas but sometimes within the UK. Primary care may be the first, and sometimes only, setting in which safe disclosure can occur.
2. **Routine consultations can uncover hidden trauma.**
   Cervical screening, contraception reviews and antenatal care are key opportunities for sensitive identification. What appears to be a routine appointment may reveal a history of profound physical and psychological harm.
3. **Observation alone is not enough – we must ask.**
   FGM is rarely disclosed spontaneously. Unless clinicians ask clearly, sensitively, and without judgement, many women will continue to suffer in silence, believing nothing can be done.
4. **Cervical screening can be re-traumatising.**
   For survivors of FGM, smear tests may be physically painful and emotionally triggering. Time, explanation, consent and the option to stop are essential to minimise harm and build trust.

5. **Know local referral pathways.**
Specialist FGM clinics offer de-infibulation, psychological support and holistic care. Primary care clinicians should be familiar with local services and confident in discussing referral options respectfully.

6. **Safeguarding responsibilities extend beyond the adult patient.**
Any disclosure of FGM should prompt consideration of safeguarding risks to younger siblings or family members. Clinicians must understand their legal duties, particularly where girls under 18 may be at risk, and follow local safeguarding procedures.

7. **One respectful question can begin healing.**
The nurse's intervention was not complex. It was calm, informed and kind. That was enough for this patient to feel acknowledged and supported for the first time. Sometimes, asking the right question at the right moment is the first step towards safety and recovery.

Reflection: Beyond the referral – listening, lifestyle and fertility

It was a busy morning clinic when I met a confident woman in her late twenties. She attended with her partner, requesting a referral to the fertility clinic. Her manner was upbeat, but beneath the smile there was a quiet undercurrent of disappointment. They had been trying to conceive for some time.

She had never carried a pregnancy to term, but she had conceived twice. Both pregnancies had ended in early miscarriage, before ten weeks. Her partner confirmed that he had never fathered a child. Both appeared physically well and were in a stable, supportive relationship.

"I'd like a referral to the fertility clinic", *she said.*

In the pace of general practice, with a ten-minute appointment and what appeared to be a clear request, it would have been easy to agree and proceed. Something made me pause. Rather than moving straight to action, I asked whether we could talk a little more before arranging the referral. She agreed.

As we explored her history further, her lifestyle emerged. Weekends were filled with hiking, climbing, cycling and travel. She lived a high-energy, physically demanding life. Behind all that vitality, I found myself wondering whether the cumulative physical strain might be playing a role, not in conception, but in sustaining an early pregnancy.

We discussed this gently, without judgement or prescription. We talked about how early pregnancy places new demands on the body, and how, for some women, it may benefit from a period of relative gentleness – prioritising rest, hydration, nutrition, and easing back from intense physical exertion in those first fragile weeks. She listened openly and thoughtfully. I reassured her that referral remained an option and that we could revisit it at any time.

Several months passed.

She returned one day with a radiant smile and a small card in her hand. She was now the mother of a healthy baby daughter. Inside the card were just a few words: "You helped me understand when I needed to slow down. Thank you for helping me become a mother".

Lessons and reflections

1. **Fertility is not only about conception.**
   Much of fertility care focuses on achieving pregnancy, yet early pregnancy loss deserves equal attention. Supporting a patient to sustain a pregnancy can require a different lens and a broader exploration.
2. **A pause for history can change everything.**
   Even in a time-pressured consultation, taking a moment to explore lifestyle, physical demands and stress can uncover modifiable factors and alter the entire direction of care.
3. **Gentle advice can have profound effects.**
   Effective guidance does not need to be forceful or directive. Thoughtful suggestions, offered with respect and humility, can be life-changing when they meet readiness and trust.
4. **Education empowers, instruction limits.**
   This was not a long consultation, but it was a meaningful one. When patients feel informed rather than told what to do, they are far more likely to engage and adapt.
5. **Look beyond the referral request.**
   A referral is often a doorway, not an endpoint. What seems like a straightforward administrative task may actually be an invitation to listen more deeply and offer care that is truly personalised.

10.8 One-liner summary

"You do not have to live with this. We have options to help you feel more in control again."

Reflective prompts:

- Think of a women's health consultation where you felt unsure or underprepared. What would you do differently now?
- How do you currently offer contraception choices? Do you begin with a list of options, or by asking what matters most to the patient?
- How comfortable do you feel discussing menopause and HRT? What is one area you would like to build confidence in?
- When a patient says, *"I've just put up with it"*, how do you respond in a way that honours her resilience while offering support?
- What language do you use to explain cycle regulation, hormone treatment or perimenopause to patients who are unsure what is happening in their bodies?

CHAPTER 11
Children and parental concerns

"You're not just treating a child, you're treating a parent's fear in ten minutes."

Paediatric consultations in general practice are short in time but long in emotion. Most childhood illnesses you see will be mild and self-limiting, yet parents rarely attend lightly. They arrive carrying a weight of worry, often built from sleepless nights, online searches, conflicting advice, and the pressure of wanting to do the right thing.

Your role is twofold: to assess the child clinically, and to manage the anxiety in the room. Sometimes the child is bouncing around the consultation room while the parent is close to tears. At other times, the child is unusually quiet, and you feel the atmosphere shift as your own concern rises.

Do not dismiss the worry. The worry is what brought them in. This chapter focuses on fever, rash, cough and the classic 'not quite right' child. It also offers practical tools for safety-netting, communication, and recognising when escalation is the safest choice.

11.1 The presentation

A 2-year-old child presents with a two-day history of fever and a new non-blanching rash. Mum is tearful. The child is tired but alert, playing intermittently, drinking fluids, and still producing wet nappies. Observations are stable.

This is the moment to step back and assess not only the rash, but the room: the parent's fear, your own clinical judgement, and the relationship between what you see and what the parent feels. A well child can present with a frightening symptom and a sick child can appear deceptively 'not too bad' at first glance.

Your task, over time, is to learn to tell the difference – and to remain safe when you cannot.

Reflection: The mid-game call that saved a life

It was a warm summer afternoon in Milton Keynes when a mother arrived at the surgery in a taxi, after pulling her 16-year-old son away from a football match. "He's not right", *she said, with quiet certainty. There were no specific complaints, just the firm conviction of a parent who sensed something others could not.*

He appeared pale but otherwise well. Calm, cooperative and polite, he reported no symptoms. There was no bleeding, no fever, and no overt signs of systemic illness. His examination was unremarkable. Yet something about his appearance, coupled with his mother's insistence, made me pause. I arranged routine blood tests that same day.

The following morning, the laboratory called.

- *Haemoglobin: 6.4g/dl*
- *Creatinine: >3000µmol/L*

I had never seen a creatinine level that high in someone so young. He was admitted immediately. Further investigations confirmed end-stage chronic kidney disease (CKD stage 5), with severe chronic anaemia secondary to erythropoietin deficiency. His illness had progressed silently, masked by youth, fitness, and remarkable physiological compensation.

Because his mother trusted her instinct, and because a simple set of blood tests was taken, he was rapidly referred to a specialist centre in London. He went on to receive a life-saving renal transplant.

Lessons and reflections

1. **Teenagers can appear well despite critical illness.**
   Adolescents often minimise symptoms, and their physiological reserves allow significant disease to remain hidden. A normal demeanour should not override clinical unease.
2. **Parental instinct matters.**
   In this case, the mother was right. Her persistence prompted investigation that may otherwise have been delayed. While not infallible, parental insight is a vital part of the clinical picture and deserves respect.
3. **Pallor is a subtle but important sign.**
   Pallor, even in isolation, warrants exploration. It may be the only outward sign of profound anaemia or chronic disease, particularly in young people who are compensating well.
4. **Simple tests can be life-saving.**
   A basic full blood count and U&Es panel revealed a catastrophic diagnosis. In general practice, so-called 'routine' tests remain among our most powerful diagnostic tools.
5. **Compensation delays diagnosis.**
   This young man's body had adapted over months, perhaps years. The absence of symptoms did not mean the absence of disease. Fitness and youth can reassure clinicians falsely if instinct is ignored.

11.2 Key questions to ask

You are looking for danger signs, but also building reassurance through structure and clarity. Key questions include:

- How long has the illness lasted, and are things improving, stable or worsening?
- Is feeding, drinking and urine output normal or reduced?
- How is the child interacting: alert, responsive and consolable, or unusually irritable, floppy or difficult to rouse?
- How high has the fever been, how long has it persisted, and does it respond to antipyretics?
- Has the rash changed, and are there associated symptoms such as breathing difficulty, vomiting or diarrhoea?
- Any sick contacts, recent travel or concerns regarding vaccination status?

Always ask: *"What are you most worried about?"*. Parental instinct is not infallible, but it is rarely meaningless. It often points to the real fear in the room and, occasionally, to the earliest sign that something is wrong.

11.3 What you must not miss

Most children are well. The risk is in the minority who are not and, in the early stages, that difference can be subtle. Be particularly alert to:

- **Meningitis**, especially with a non-blanching rash, altered consciousness, neck stiffness or photophobia.
- **Sepsis**, suggested by lethargy, pallor, poor perfusion, reduced feeding, capillary refill time >2 seconds, or a very high or unusually low heart rate.
- **Urinary tract infection** in infants, particularly fever without a clear focus.
- **Bronchiolitis, croup or epiglottitis**, especially in babies under six months or any child with stridor or signs of respiratory distress.
- **Parental concern**, especially when a parent states, "*They are just not right*", even if objective signs appear borderline.

You will not always be certain, but you can always be safe: discuss early with a senior colleague, arrange review, and escalate when needed. The aim is not perfection, it is safety.

11.4 The likely reality

In everyday practice:

- Most febrile illnesses in under-fives are viral and self-limiting.
- Non-blanching rashes are often petechiae from coughing, vomiting or minor pressure, or can occur with viral illness, but they must always be taken seriously.

Reflection: Limping in a war zone – the courage to act

She was 9 years old, limping, febrile and visibly unwell. She complained of deep, persistent pain in her left thigh. There had been no trauma, no insect bites, and no obvious cause – yet something was clearly wrong.

She had been referred from the outpatient department to the minor operations area. Her temperature was raised and her heart rate was high. Her small body was responding to something hidden and potentially serious. Clinical instinct suggested this was more than a superficial infection. The possibility of necrotising fasciitis lingered quietly but firmly in my mind.

It was after 4 o'clock in the afternoon in Muthur, a small peninsula town in the war-affected northeast of Sri Lanka. Transfer to the nearest base hospital was not possible. Roads were unsafe after dark due to landmines. Sea routes were dangerous, and air evacuation was not available. At that moment, there was no higher level of care. There was only what we could do with the resources at hand.

I explained the situation carefully to her father and obtained consent. Under local anaesthesia, I inserted a wide-bore needle into the mid-thigh. Within seconds, the syringe filled with pus. A deep abscess had been draining into the surrounding tissues. This confirmed a serious infection and, just as importantly, reduced the likelihood of a far more catastrophic diagnosis.

She was kept under close observation overnight. By morning, she was stable enough for safe transfer to Trincomalee Base Hospital, where the surgical team continued her care. She was out of immediate danger.

This was not simply a case of a child with a limp. It was a moment where medical urgency collided with geopolitical reality. In that setting, a bedside needle aspiration was not only appropriate, it was essential. This experience stands as a tribute to clinicians working at the limits of possibility, where courage, judgement and compassion must substitute for infrastructure.

Lessons and reflections

1. **Necrotising fasciitis must be considered early.**
   Deep limb pain combined with systemic features should always prompt concern for serious infection. Early investigation and decisive action can be life-saving, even before overt skin changes appear.
2. **Needle aspiration can provide critical answers.**
   When access to imaging or theatre is limited, bedside aspiration can offer immediate diagnostic clarity and guide urgent management decisions.
3. **Use ultrasound when available.**
   In better-resourced environments, ultrasound improves accuracy, helps localise collections, and can reduce unnecessary delay or tissue trauma.
4. **Physiology often speaks louder than history.**
   The absence of trauma does not exclude danger. Fever, tachycardia and an unwell appearance in a child warrant prompt escalation and investigation.

5. **Resourcefulness is a clinical skill.**
   Practising medicine in conflict zones demands adaptability and moral courage. When technology is absent, careful examination and sound clinical judgement become the most powerful tools available.

- Parents often apologise for 'wasting your time'. Your response matters: validate their decision to attend and reinforce that seeking assessment was appropriate.

A calm, confident tone can settle a frightened parent more effectively than any leaflet, particularly when paired with a clear plan.

11.5 What to do

Fever with likely viral symptoms

- Assess hydration carefully: wet nappies, tears, mucous membranes, skin turgor and overall activity.
- Record vital signs, including heart rate, respiratory rate, capillary refill time, oxygen saturations and temperature.
- Consider urine testing and culture in infants or young children with fever and no obvious source.
- Reassure when the child is alert, hydrated and clinically improving, while clearly explaining what to monitor and when to seek help.

Non-blanching rash

- Perform a full and careful examination, including skin folds, scalp and mucous membranes.
- Repeat observations if needed; do not anchor your decision on a single set of vital signs.
- Escalate if you are unsure. It is safer to discuss early with paediatrics than to sit with doubt.

Good paediatric care is not just recognising the unwell child; it is also recognising when you need support to make a safe decision.

11.6 Safety-netting advice

Be crystal clear. Repeat key points. Write them down where possible. Parents are often exhausted, anxious and unlikely to retain everything you say.

Examples of clear safety-netting include:

- *"If they become harder to wake, start breathing faster, stop weeing as normal, or if the rash spreads or changes, please seek urgent help."*
- *"Even if nothing has changed but you are still worried, come back. We would rather see you again than miss something."*

Safety-netting is not an afterthought. It is part of the treatment plan.

Reflection: The knee pain that meant more – a missed opportunity for early detection

He was 11 years old and brought in by his mother with a sore throat. The consultation was straightforward. As they were leaving, his mother paused at the door and said, "By the way, doctor, he's been complaining of pain in his right knee. But at this age they say all sorts of things to get out of school, so I wouldn't worry".

I offered to arrange another appointment to assess his knee properly, but his mother declined, reassuring me that it was not necessary. I carried out a brief examination to decide whether the consultation needed to be extended. There were no obvious red flags. There was no swelling, no history of trauma, no limp, and nothing to suggest infection or acute injury. I provided reassurance, supportive advice and safety-netting.

That consultation took place in April.

In August, his name appeared again, this time on the triage list, with a history of limping. I recognised him from our brief encounter months earlier and arranged an urgent same-day appointment. Imaging and subsequent biopsy confirmed the diagnosis of osteosarcoma.

Despite treatment, he died peacefully at the age of 16.

Later, his mother expressed deep regret that she had not taken his early complaints more seriously. For me, this case has never faded. It remains a reminder that what presents as an aside, a fleeting comment, or a seemingly minor symptom may, on rare occasions, be the earliest sign of something life-changing.

Lessons and reflections

1. **Children's symptoms deserve careful attention.**
   Even when parents downplay concerns, new or unexplained symptoms in children warrant deliberate consideration. Children rely on adults to take their experiences seriously.
2. **Knee pain is usually benign, but not always.**
   Most childhood musculoskeletal pain is self-limiting. Occasionally, persistent or unexplained pain can be an early sign of serious pathology, including malignancy. Although rare, it matters.
3. **Parents often minimise out of reassurance, not neglect.**
   Many parents normalise symptoms in an effort to reassure themselves or their child. Our role is to listen carefully, explore gently, and balance reassurance with appropriate vigilance.
4. **Safety-netting sometimes needs planned follow-up.**
   Advice to return if symptoms persist is essential. In selected cases, particularly involving children, planned review or active recall may help prevent delayed diagnosis.
5. **Some cases stay with us, and they should.**
   Not every poor outcome reflects an error, but some encounters shape how we practise forever. They sharpen our awareness, deepen our listening, and remind us to stay alert to subtle signs, however minor they may seem.

Reflection: When waiting costs more than we realise

He was 7 when I first met him, brought in by parents who were unsure how to begin. There was no single dramatic concern, no crisis moment that forced the appointment. Instead, there was a collection of small worries that had been quietly accumulating over time. He struggled to sit still. He found transitions difficult. His emotional responses seemed bigger than the situations that triggered them. At school, he was falling behind in ways that did not quite fit with his intelligence.

At home, his parents had adapted. They had learnt his patterns, anticipated his reactions, softened routines, and explained things repeatedly. Like many families, they told themselves he would grow out of it. Children develop at different speeds, after all. They did not want to label him. They did not want to make a fuss.

The school had raised gentle concerns. Nothing urgent, just observations. Difficulty with attention. Social challenges. Emotional dysregulation. Again, nothing dramatic enough to force action. Time passed.

By the time he came to see me, his confidence had begun to erode. He knew he was different, even if he did not have the words for it. He was starting to believe that the problem was him. His parents, now more anxious than hesitant, wondered aloud whether they had waited too long.

The consultation was not about diagnosis. It was about listening. About recognising patterns that were already there. The possibility of neurodiversity had been present for years, but it had remained unnamed, unaddressed and therefore unsupported.

We spoke about next steps. The role of the GP. The importance of the school SENCo. The value of early assessment, even when the pathway feels slow and uncertain. I reassured them that seeking help was not a failure, and that recognising neurodiversity is not about limiting a child, but about understanding them.

What stayed with me was not the complexity of the case, but the quiet grief that often accompanies delayed recognition. Not because parents do not care, but because they hope. They wait. They normalise. And in doing so, they sometimes lose precious time.

Lessons and reflections

1. **Early signs deserve early attention.**
   Difficulties with attention, emotional regulation, communication or social interaction should not be dismissed simply because they are subtle or variable. Patterns matter more than single behaviours.

2. **Waiting rarely makes neurodiversity disappear.**
   Children do not grow out of autism, ADHD, or related neurodevelopmental differences. What they often grow into is misunderstanding, frustration, and reduced self-esteem if support is delayed.

3. **Parents are not overreacting by asking questions.**
   Raising concerns early is not about labelling a child. It is about opening doors to understanding, adjustments, and support at home and at school.

4. **Schools and GPs must work together.**
   SENCos, teachers and primary care clinicians each see different parts of the child's world. When concerns are shared early, the picture becomes clearer and the pathway smoother.
5. **Delay has a cost.**
   Missed support in the early years can affect education, mental health, family relationships and long-term outcomes. What is lost is not just time, but confidence and opportunity.
6. **Recognition is an act of care.**
   Naming neurodiversity does not reduce a child's potential. It protects it. Understanding how a child's brain works allows us to build environments where they can thrive.

11.7 What I wish I had known

You will not always see textbook presentations. Much of paediatrics in primary care involves blending observation, parental instinct and your own clinical judgement. Stay calm, speak slowly and treat the concern seriously.

You may not always be right. But if you are safe, transparent and communicative, you will not be careless.

You are not just managing illness, you are managing fear, trust and time.

11.8 One-liner summary

"Things look reassuring right now, but if anything changes or you are worried again, please do not hesitate to come back."

Reflective prompts:

- When was the last time you felt unsure in a paediatric consultation? What did you do, and what did you learn from it?
- How do you balance your clinical assessment with parental instinct when the two do not align?
- Think of a time you gave safety-netting advice to a parent. What words did you choose, and how did they respond?
- How do you maintain your composure when a parent is visibly distressed or overwhelmed?
- What physical signs or instincts do you rely on most when deciding whether a child is well enough to go home?

CHAPTER 12
Sleep, fatigue and 'generally unwell'

"Just because it is vague does not mean it is harmless. But it also does not always mean disease."

"Tired all the time." "Run down." "Can't concentrate." These phrases appear in general practice every day. They often point not to a single diagnosis, but to a complex intersection of physical, psychological and social factors. Fatigue and vague unwellness may arise from minor deficiencies, poor sleep, low mood, chronic stress, or simply the cumulative weight of life feeling overwhelming.

The challenge lies in taking the symptom seriously without over-investigating or dismissing the person's experience. Fatigue is never 'just tiredness'; there is always a story behind it. This chapter aims to help you feel more confident working with uncertainty and building clear, supportive care plans, even when an immediate answer is not available.

12.1 The presentation

A 38-year-old woman presents with several months of fatigue. She reports no pain and no fever. Her sleep is fragmented. She is juggling work alongside caring for young children. *"It's probably nothing,"* she says, *"but I'm fed up."*

When patients describe symptoms this vague, their fatigue is genuine, and so is their frustration. Even when examination is unremarkable and investigations return as normal, your words, explanations and follow-up plan still matter greatly.

12.2 Key questions to ask

Your questions often uncover more than your blood request forms ever will. Key areas to explore include:

- When did the fatigue begin, and was the onset sudden or gradual?
- What impact is it having on daily life, including work, parenting, motivation and enjoyment?

Reflection: The quiet concern – when family sees what the patient does not

It was a warm morning in the Australian outback when a 76-year-old man attended with his wife. He appeared calm and even cheerful, but it was his wife who spoke first. "He's just not himself", *she said gently.* "He's tired all the time. He won't admit it, but I can see it."

When I asked how he was feeling, he smiled and brushed it aside, "I'm fine. Just getting old" *he said. He mentioned some mild lower back pain, which he dismissed as insignificant. His examination was unremarkable. There were no obvious red flags and no immediate cause for concern. Even so, a quiet sense of unease remained. Experience has taught me that partners often notice changes long before clinicians do.*

I arranged blood tests, extending beyond the routine panel to include inflammatory markers. When the results returned, his erythrocyte sedimentation rate was 70mm per hour and his globulin levels were raised. Something was sitting behind the fatigue he had not voiced. I proceeded to request a myeloma screen, including serum protein electrophoresis, immunoglobulins, and urine testing for light chains.

Within days, the diagnosis was confirmed. He had multiple myeloma. Because the condition was identified at an earlier stage, he was referred promptly to haematology and treatment was initiated before irreversible complications developed. His wife's quiet concern had changed the course of his illness.

Lessons and reflections

1. **Family observations matter.**
   Those closest to a patient often detect subtle changes that are not immediately apparent in the consultation room. Even understated comments should be taken seriously.
2. **Patients frequently minimise symptoms.**
   Older adults, in particular, may normalise fatigue, pain or slowing down as part of ageing. It is our role to pause and consider when these changes warrant further exploration.
3. **Blood tests can reveal what history does not.**
   Raised inflammatory markers and abnormal globulin levels, even without dramatic symptoms, should prompt further investigation. In conditions such as myeloma, early biochemical clues are crucial.
4. **Use collective clinical wisdom.**
   Discussing uncertain cases with colleagues can clarify thinking and strengthen decision-making. General practice is safer and more effective when it is collaborative.
5. **Curiosity strengthens good clinical practice.**
   Guidelines provide structure, but patients do not always fit neatly within them. A small step beyond the obvious, one extra question or one additional test, can sometimes be the difference between delay and timely diagnosis.

- What is sleep like in practice: quality, duration, interruptions and patterns?
- Are there changes in mood, appetite and anxiety levels, or loss of interest?
- Are there red flags such as unintentional weight loss, night sweats, bleeding or persistent pain?
- Is there relevant medical history, including menstrual patterns, thyroid disease, previous anaemia or chronic illness?
- What is the broader context: work stress, burnout, caring responsibilities, recent loss or major life changes?

These questions help you build a narrative rather than a checklist – and allow the patient to feel seen rather than processed.

12.3 What you must not miss

Certain causes of fatigue require active exclusion. Always keep in mind:

- Anaemia, particularly in people with heavy menstrual bleeding or iron-poor diets.
- Thyroid disease, especially in those with autoimmune risk or during the postpartum period.
- Coeliac disease, particularly where gastrointestinal symptoms or family history are present.
- Depression and anxiety, which are common, disabling and highly treatable.
- Malignancy, rare but important, especially when accompanied by weight loss, night sweats or persistent pain.
- Obstructive sleep apnoea, particularly in individuals who snore, are overweight, and report excessive daytime sleepiness.

The aim is not to investigate everything, but to miss nothing important.

12.4 The likely reality

In most cases:

- Fatigue is multifactorial, involving a blend of sleep disruption, stress, mood changes, lifestyle factors and minor deficiencies.
- Many patients harbour unspoken fears of serious disease, even if they minimise their symptoms aloud.
- Even when no single unifying diagnosis emerges, you can still meaningfully improve quality of life.

You do not always need a definitive diagnosis to make a difference.

12.5 What to do

Initial investigations (first presentation in adults)

- Consider a baseline panel such as full blood count, ferritin, TFTs, HbA1c, LFTs, U&Es, vitamin B12, folate, ESR and bone profile, tailoring to history and local guidance.
- Add vitamin D, coeliac screening, or more detailed iron studies when the clinical context suggests increased risk.

For children

- Adapt investigations to age and presentation. This may include full blood count, inflammatory markers, vitamin D and a random glucose, alongside targeted tests guided by symptoms and examination.

Sleep-related concerns

- Explore caffeine intake, evening screen use, shift work and irregular sleep patterns.
- Offer clear sleep hygiene advice and, where available, signpost to cognitive behavioural therapy for insomnia (CBT-i) or structured self-help resources.
- Reserve short-term pharmacological sleep aids for situations where function is significantly impaired and non-pharmacological measures have failed, and ensure prompt review.

Non-specific fatigue

- Validate the symptom explicitly and acknowledge that fatigue is real, even when tests are normal.
- Explore stressors, coping strategies and sources of support.
- Avoid prematurely medicalising everyday pressures, but do not minimise genuine distress.
- Arrange a follow-up appointment in four to six weeks to review progress, discuss results and agree on next steps together.

Structure and follow-up often matter more than any single intervention.

12.6 Safety-netting advice

Clarity and contingency planning are essential. Examples include:

- *"If you lose weight without trying, develop night sweats, or feel persistently more unwell, please return promptly rather than waiting until next week."*
- *"Normal blood results are reassuring, but if your symptoms continue or worsen, we will review this again and adjust our plan."*

A planned review can be more therapeutic than a rushed referral.

Reflection: The midnight numbness – unravelling severe vitamin B12 deficiency

It was the early 2000s in Milton Keynes when a young woman in her mid-twenties came to see me. She looked worn down and slightly apologetic as she described a familiar complaint. She was tired all the time.

She was working long shifts at a fast food outlet and living in poor conditions in the flat above. Her diet, she admitted, consisted largely of leftover takeaway food, with chips and fried meals most days.

One detail made me pause. She described numbness in both feet, particularly at night. It was not painful, but it was persistent and unusual. There were no other neurological signs on examination. In another context, this might easily have been attributed to fatigue, lifestyle or footwear.

With the help of our healthcare assistant, who kindly fitted her in for blood tests between patients, we were able to investigate further.

Her results were striking. Her serum vitamin B12 level was almost undetectable, and her mean corpuscular volume was 122. We had identified the problem just in time. She was admitted to hospital immediately.

The story then took an unexpected turn. The admitting consultant, who had previously worked extensively in Africa, chose to administer vitamin B12 intravenously rather than via the usual intramuscular route. Based on his experience, he believed this would achieve a faster systemic response. He was right.

Her improvement was dramatic. Within days, the numbness began to resolve. Her energy levels improved and her mood lifted. What could have progressed to permanent neurological damage was reversed, simply because someone had paused, listened carefully, and acted early.

Lessons and reflections

1. **Fatigue in young adults should not be dismissed.**
   Tiredness in younger people is often attributed to stress, overwork or lifestyle. When fatigue is accompanied by neurological symptoms such as numbness or tingling, further investigation is essential.
2. **Vitamin B12 deficiency can be insidious and severe.**
   With a markedly raised mean corpuscular volume and near-absent vitamin B12 levels, this patient was at real risk of subacute combined degeneration. Early recognition changed the outcome entirely.
3. **Varied clinical experience strengthens decision-making.**
   The consultant's prior experience in resource-limited settings informed an unconventional but effective treatment choice. Exposure to diverse healthcare systems can broaden clinical thinking and improve patient care.
4. **Teamwork prevents harm.**
   If the blood test had not been taken that day, this diagnosis may have been delayed. Small acts of flexibility and cooperation within the primary care team can prevent serious long-term consequences.

5. **Nutrition is a core clinical issue.**
   This patient was not overtly malnourished, but her diet lacked essential nutrients over time. Asking about what people actually eat is an important diagnostic step, not a social aside.
6. **Early treatment protects neurological function.**
   Once neurological symptoms of vitamin B12 deficiency develop, delay increases the risk of permanent damage. Timely intervention can mean the difference between recovery and lifelong disability.

12.7 What I wish I had known

You do not need a definitive diagnosis to provide excellent care. A patient who leaves feeling heard, believed, and with a clear next step has already benefited.

Listening is powerful. It communicates care, often more effectively than medication.

12.8 One-liner summary

"There may not be a single clear cause, but we will take this seriously and work through it together, step by step."

Reflective prompts:

- Think of a time you ordered a full blood panel for fatigue. What was the outcome, and how clinically useful was it?
- How do you approach vague presentations to avoid both over-investigation and under-validation?
- What language do you use when there is no obvious diagnosis, but the patient still feels unwell?
- How do you manage your own emotional reserves during multiple 'general tiredness' consultations in a single day?
- When a patient felt genuinely heard despite not receiving tests or medication, how did you know it had landed well? What did they say or do?

CHAPTER 13

Reflections from the consulting room

Reflection: D-dimer at dusk – the Friday that didn't let me go

It was just after 6.30 pm, the close of another long duty doctor day. My notes were finished, my coat was on, and I was already halfway home in my head, thinking about dinner. Any GP who has done enough duty days knows that quiet end-of-day hope. Please, no more calls.

That Friday evening, the phone rang.

Reception put through a call from the hospital laboratory. They said it was an urgent result. I felt that familiar tightening in my chest. A 57-year-old man. Left leg swelling. His D-dimer had come back at 7000.

I opened his notes. He had been seen earlier by one of our salaried GPs. Concerned about a possible DVT, she had ordered the blood test. Sensible reasoning in the moment. But now the DVT clinic was closed. The result was here. And the responsibility had landed with me.

I phoned the patient. No answer.

I tried again. Still nothing.

I called a third time, now acutely aware of how much depended on this conversation. Eventually, after what felt far longer than it was, he picked up. I explained the result, the concern, and the need to be assessed urgently. He listened carefully and agreed to go straight to A&E.

There were no sirens. No dramatic collapse in the waiting room. Just a quiet escalation that could easily have gone unseen. A moment that passed almost unnoticed, yet one that could have ended very differently.

That is the nature of general practice. Sometimes it is not the dramatic cases that stay with you, but the ordinary ones that nearly slip away.

Lessons and reflections

1. **Do not use D-dimer in primary care to rule out DVT.**
   If the clinical suspicion of DVT is high enough to order a D-dimer, it is high enough to refer. A raised result late on a Friday, with no service to act on it, creates risk rather than reassurance.

2. **Every test ordered is a clinical commitment.**
   Blood tests are not administrative tasks. They are decisions that carry responsibility. There must always be a clear plan for how results will be reviewed and acted upon.
3. **Be wary of the weekend gap.**
   Results do not respect surgery hours. Before ordering an urgent test on a Friday, ask yourself who will see the result and what will happen if it is abnormal.
4. **Once you see the result, it is yours.**
   It is tempting to rationalise delay or assume someone else will pick it up. But once a result is known, responsibility cannot be deferred. Patient safety depends on follow-through.
5. **Reflection should change practice.**
   After this case, we discussed it as a team and changed our approach. No D-dimers for suspected DVT in primary care. If the concern is there, the referral should be too. Clear, simple and safer for everyone.

Reflection: When the note wasn't enough

Sometimes, it is not a patient's symptoms that raise concern, but what sits quietly in the background. This case came to my attention during a routine review of outstanding clinical queries, the sort of task that rarely feels urgent until it suddenly is.

Buried in the record was a chest X-ray report from several weeks earlier. The radiologist had recommended a course of antibiotics and a repeat chest X-ray in six weeks. Sensible advice. The GP who had reviewed the result had added a brief note: "Follow-up with a clinician needed."

And that was where the story paused. No follow-up had been arranged. No appointment booked. No task created. Nothing had moved.

When I spoke to the GP, he was genuinely taken aback. He had assumed that adding the note would prompt the administrative team to act. In his mind, the intention was clear. In reality, the system did nothing with it. This was not carelessness or avoidance. It was a misunderstanding of how our local processes worked. He was new to the practice and had not yet learnt which actions required explicit tasking, and which did not.

Thankfully, the patient remained well. Once the gap was identified, we contacted him, arranged the follow-up imaging, and brought the episode back on track. Continuity was restored without harm.

But it did not sit easily. Not because something had gone wrong, but because it so nearly had.

This was a reminder that in modern general practice, safety often depends less on clinical knowledge and more on how well we understand the systems that sit around it. Good intentions alone do not move care forward. Actions do.

Lessons and reflections

1. **Notes are not actions.**
   Documenting a thought does not make it happen. If follow-up is required, it must be linked to a clear and traceable action, whether that is a task to admin, a booked appointment, or a clinician reminder.
2. **Do not assume the system understands your intent.**
   Electronic records can give a false sense of reassurance. Unless a note is connected to a defined workflow, it remains passive. Knowing how your system behaves is as important as knowing what to write.
3. **Induction matters more than we realise.**
   Even experienced GPs need proper onboarding when joining a new practice. Every system has its own rhythms, shortcuts and risks. Safety depends on understanding them early.
4. **Reflection should strengthen safety, not assign blame.**
   This case was recorded as a Significant Event Analysis. The GP engaged fully, reflected honestly, and committed to auditing his follow-ups. That response improves care far more than defensiveness ever could.
5. **Chance is not a safety strategy.**
   This gap was identified through routine review, not because the system flagged it. Follow-up plans should not rely on luck. Regular checks and clear processes protect both patients and clinicians.

Reflection: The missed value

It began as a routine triage task. Parents had requested a follow-up appointment to discuss their daughter's blood results. She was almost 14 years old. The GP who had reviewed the full blood count had sent an automated message advising a routine appointment within two weeks. On the surface, everything appeared appropriate.

But something did not sit comfortably.

When I opened the results myself, all parameters were within normal range, except for one which stood out immediately. Her haemoglobin was 73g/L; not the MCV, not a borderline result, her haemoglobin.

In any patient, that value matters. In a young adolescent who had already reported tiredness, dizziness and a fainting episode, it was a clear red flag. I arranged a same-day consultation and made a conscious decision to follow the case through personally.

Later that evening, before logging off, I checked the record again. What I found was unsettling. There had been one attempt to contact the family. No answer. The entry stopped there. No further plan documented.

I called the family myself. Her father answered. He told me she was not cur-

rently menstruating, but that she had been experiencing heavy periods for some time. She was pale, exhausted and increasingly unwell. This was not a case for reassurance or oral iron alone. I referred her directly to the Paediatric Assessment Unit for urgent review.

In the days that followed, two important conversations took place. The GP who had initially reviewed the blood results realised that he had misread the haemoglobin value as MCV. It was an honest mistake, but a significant one. The second doctor, overwhelmed by the pressures of the day, had not made further attempts to contact the family after the first call went unanswered.

This was not a catastrophe. But it was uncomfortably close.

What stayed with me was how easily the outcome could have been different. A single misread value, followed by an assumption that someone else would pick things up, nearly resulted in a dangerous delay. It was a reminder that our safety-nets are only as strong as the systems and habits that support them.

Lessons and reflections

1. **Misreading can happen to anyone.**
   Confusing haemoglobin with MCV is an easy and potentially dangerous error, particularly under pressure. In children and adolescents, critical values must always prompt direct clinician action rather than automated advice.
2. **Automated communication has limits.**
   Text messages and electronic follow-ups have their place, but they cannot replace direct contact when results are abnormal or urgent.
3. **Triage is a clinical responsibility.**
   Triage is not administrative work. It is a protective clinical role that allows missed concerns to be identified and corrected.
4. **One unanswered call is not enough.**
   When results are critical, failure to make contact must trigger escalation. Silence should never be an endpoint.
5. **Systems must anticipate human error.**
   Following this case, we reviewed how abnormal results are flagged and followed up. Safety alerts, tasking systems and second reviews all exist to catch inevitable human mistakes.
6. **Openness strengthens safety.**
   Both clinicians responded with honesty and reflection. This was not about blame, but about learning. A culture that allows mistakes to be acknowledged is one that genuinely protects patients.

PART 3

SURVIVING GP TRAINING

"You're not just learning medicine. You're learning to be a GP – and that's a different kind of training."

CHAPTER 14
The first clinic

"You're about to sit in the GP chair. It swivels, it squeaks – and soon, it will feel like home."

Your first GP clinic session is often one of the most quietly disorientating moments of your training. One minute, you are observing from the corner of a room, listening, watching, learning how others hold uncertainty. The next, you are sitting alone at a desk, door closed, with a list of names on a screen and the unspoken expectation that you will begin.

There is no announcement to mark this transition. No clear signal that something important has shifted. General practice does not dramatise its milestones. It simply opens the door, places you in the chair, and trusts that you will find your way.

This chapter is not about knowing what to do. It is about learning how to be, in that room, in that role, in those early consultations where confidence is tentative and responsibility feels newly tangible.

14.1 Walking into the room

The first consultation feels oddly formal and strangely intimate at the same time.

You walk into a small room, close the door, and suddenly realise the patient is looking directly at you. Not past you. Not waiting for someone else to arrive. Just you.

Introduce yourself clearly, even if they assume you are 'the doctor'. Say their name, smile, sit upright and face them.

These small actions matter more than you might realise. They create steadiness at a moment when you may not yet feel it internally.

If the moment feels awkward, that is entirely normal. Patients are used to new faces – trainees rotate constantly – and most are generous with their patience. What they respond to is not polish or certainty, but presence.

Be there. Listen without rushing. Allow pauses, and let the consultation breathe.

In general practice, confidence rarely comes from certainty. It comes from attentiveness.

14.2 Sitting in the chair

There is a particular second, often unnoticed, when you first sit in the GP chair and realise that something has changed.

The chair swivels. It squeaks. It may feel slightly too low or too high. But it carries weight.

From this chair, you will reassure and escalate. You will hesitate, decide, revisit, and occasionally surprise yourself. You will carry other people's worries while quietly managing your own.

At first, the role may feel borrowed, as though you are temporarily occupying someone else's position. Over time, it will begin to feel familiar.

This is not a dramatic transformation. It happens slowly, almost imperceptibly, through repetition and reflection.

14.3 Navigating the systems (without letting them take over)

Alongside the patient, the other silent presence in the room is the computer.

EMIS or SystmOne will feel clunky, unintuitive and occasionally unforgiving. You will worry about clicking the wrong option, missing an alert, or losing your place mid-consultation. This anxiety is part of early training.

At this stage, focus only on what you need to function safely:

- Coding a consultation clearly
- Requesting blood tests
- Generating referrals
- Issuing or amending sick notes.

Ask your administrative team for help. They often understand the system better than anyone else and can save you hours of frustration if you let them.

Templates and shortcuts will come later. Tools such as Ardens can be useful, but do not rush to optimise before you understand how your practice actually works.

Systems matter, but they should never dominate the consultation. If the screen becomes a barrier, pause. Turn back to the patient and reconnect.

14.4 The shock of pace

You will overrun. Almost everyone does. Ten minutes feels impossibly short when you are trying to listen properly, think safely, document clearly, and make decisions you can stand by. It is tempting to measure yourself by how quickly you clear your list, but resist that urge.

Early on, focus on one good consultation at a time. If something does not feel right, then pause. Ask for help. Bring the patient back. Speak to your supervisor mid-consult if needed. This is not incompetence. It is the practice of safe medicine.

Your job is not to get through the list. Your job is to look after the person in front of you.

Speed arrives later. Judgement comes first.

14.5 Asking for help is part of the role

When you sit alone in that room, you may feel pressure to prove that you belong there. You do not need to. Asking for help is not a failure of independence. It is a core professional skill. Thoughtful questions demonstrate insight, not weakness.

Most supervisors would far rather hear: "*Can I run something past you?*" than "*I've got no idea what I'm doing*". The first invites collaboration. The second invites rescue.

As a trainer and appraiser, I have never been concerned about trainees who asked for advice. I have worried about those who did not.

14.6 Living with the fear

Imposter syndrome often arrives early and lingers quietly. You may feel it when you close the consulting room door, when you send your first referral, when a patient looks unconvinced by your explanation, or when you replay a consultation long after the clinic ends. This does not mean you are failing. It means you care.

Breathe. Write things down. Ask early. Reflect later.

One day, often without noticing exactly when, you will realise the chair feels familiar. Patterns will emerge, explanations will simplify, and patients will ask to see you again.

Growth in general practice is gradual, subtle and mostly invisible from the inside.

14.7 What I wish I had known

I wish I had known that it is acceptable not to love general practice immediately. You do not have to feel like a GP on day one, or even in the first few months. The role grows around you. Confidence settles quietly. Belonging comes later.

Every GP you admire has sat in that same chair, unsure, watching the clock, wondering if they were doing enough.

You are not behind. You are exactly where you are meant to be.

Final thought

The first time you sit alone in the GP chair, nothing dramatic happens. The room is quiet. The screen flickers. A patient waits.

And yet something important has shifted.

You are no longer just learning medicine. You are beginning to carry it, thoughtfully, imperfectly, and with care. This is how general practice is learnt: not through sudden confidence, but through small, steady acts of presence, repeated day after day.

Reflective prompts:

- What did it feel like the first time you closed the consulting room door on your own?
- Which part of the consultation felt most unfamiliar: the responsibility, the uncertainty, or being seen as 'the GP'?
- When did you notice yourself trying to sound more confident than you felt? What helped in that moment?
- Who did you reach out to after your early clinics, and what support mattered most?
- What would you like your future self to remember about these first days?

CHAPTER 15

How to approach your first few clinics

"You don't have to be fast. You have to be safe, kind and curious."

Your first few clinics as a GP trainee are unlikely to feel smooth, efficient or neatly contained within the timetable. They will almost certainly run over. You may finish with a long list of notes still to type, unanswered questions lingering in your mind, and the quiet refrain of *"Should I have...?"* following you home.

That is not a sign that you are struggling. It is a sign that you are learning.

The aim at this stage is not perfection. It is to begin finding your rhythm, developing clinical judgement, and noticing the small wins hidden within the apparent chaos of early practice.

15.1 It's not a performance – it's a process

In the early days, many trainees feel as though each consultation is an audition: for their trainer, for the patient, and often for themselves. There is a sense of being watched, measured and quietly assessed.

But general practice is not a performance.

Patients are not looking for polish. They are looking for presence. They want to feel listened to, taken seriously, and gently guided through uncertainty. They want someone who can sit with complexity without rushing to conclusions.

Your task is not to impress. It is to be present, prepared and human.

If you leave a consultation knowing the patient felt heard and understood, you have done something important, even if the plan felt imperfect.

15.2 Plan for slowness

If you are given longer appointment slots at the start of training, possibly twenty or even thirty minutes, use them fully and without apology. This time is not indulgence; it is investment.

Early clinics are where you learn how to:

- Take a structured but flexible history
- Think aloud and explain uncertainty clearly
- Look up guidance safely and transparently
- Write notes that reflect reasoning, not just outcomes
- Discuss cases with your supervisor while they are still fresh.

Soon enough, ten-minute appointments will arrive. When they do, the habits you build now – how you listen, how you prioritise, how you pause – will matter far more than speed ever could.

Slowness at the beginning is not inefficiency. It is how safe clinicians are formed.

15.3 Document with your future self in mind

One day, you will read your own notes again. It may be later that afternoon, weeks later, or years down the line. Write them for that future version of you. Good documentation is not defensive; it is thoughtful.

Helpful habits include:

- Recording red flags you actively considered and excluded
- Documenting safety-netting clearly and explicitly
- Writing a brief summary at the top of the record (for example: '32-year-old female, headache 5 days, no red flags, likely migraine')
- Noting what you explained, what was agreed, and what happens next.

Well-written notes are more than a record. They are a safety-net, for your patient and for you.

15.4 Flag uncertainty – then follow it up

Uncertainty is unavoidable in general practice. What matters is what you do with it.

If something feels unresolved, name it. Make a note. Return to it later. Learning on the job is not risky when it is paired with reflection and follow-up. This may mean:

- Checking NICE guidance or GPnotebook after clinic
- Discussing a case briefly with your supervisor
- Bringing a question to your next tutorial
- Reviewing outcomes when the patient returns.

Learning does not always happen in the room. Often, it happens just after.

Responsibility is not about knowing everything. It is about recognising what you do not yet know and acting on it.

15.5 Build a post-clinic routine

Early clinics can feel draining because they end abruptly. One moment you are deep in decision-making; the next, you are expected to move on.

A simple post-clinic routine can make a significant difference. This might include:

- A few quiet minutes to breathe and reset
- Jotting down questions you want to revisit
- A brief conversation with your supervisor
- A short checklist of unresolved tasks or learning points.

Turning each clinic into a moment of reflection, rather than endurance, helps training feel purposeful rather than exhausting.

15.6 What I wish I had known

I wish I had understood earlier that feeling behind does not mean you *are* behind. Early GP training is cognitively heavy. You are learning medicine, systems, relationships and risk management all at once.

You do not need to master everything immediately. You need to keep showing up, thinking carefully and asking honest questions. That is how a GP is formed.

Final thought

Your first clinics are not an exam. They are a training ground. You will not get everything right. You will miss things, run late and replay consultations in your head. And yet, with every patient, every note, and every honest conversation about what felt difficult, something important is taking shape.

This is where you begin building your GP mind – one patient, one question, one careful decision at a time.

Reflective prompts:

- What felt hardest about your first few clinics, and what helped most in that moment?
- How do you respond internally when you start running behind schedule?
- Think of an early consultation you would approach differently now. What has changed?
- How do you keep track of learning points without becoming overwhelmed?
- What kind of GP do you hope to be six months from now, and what small habits could move you closer to that?

CHAPTER 16
Ten minutes at a time

"The art of general practice is knowing what to focus on, and what to leave for another day."

The ten-minute consultation is central to life in general practice, but it is often misunderstood. It is neither a rigid deadline nor a fixed script. Patients do not arrive neatly packaged, and consultations rarely unfold in a linear way. The challenge is not to force reality into ten minutes, but to use structure thoughtfully so that care, clarity and safety remain possible under pressure.

When structure is treated as a guide rather than a template, it creates space rather than restriction. It allows you to listen, prioritise and plan, even when time feels tight. This chapter is about learning to work with ten minutes, not fighting against it.

16.1 Structure is freedom

Starting with structure does not diminish empathy. It enhances it.

A strong opening question sets the tone for the whole consultation. Asking "*What brought you in today?*" centres the patient's agenda immediately. It signals that they are being listened to and that their concern matters. It also gives you a clearer starting point, which helps you use time more effectively.

Early exploration of ideas, concerns and expectations brings depth without length. Asking "*What do you think might be going on?*", "*What's worrying you most?*" and "*What were you hoping we might do today?*" reveals not only the clinical problem but the emotional and cognitive landscape surrounding it. This information often saves time later by preventing misunderstandings or unmet expectations.

Red-flag questioning can be woven in calmly and transparently. A simple explanation such as "*I'm going to ask a few questions just to make sure there's nothing more serious going on*" reassures patients without alarming them and reinforces your role as a safe clinician.

Summarising mid-consultation is one of the most powerful time-management tools available. Saying *"so what I'm hearing is..."* confirms shared understanding, highlights priorities, and creates a natural transition into examination or planning.

Structure should never feel rigid. Some consultations need space for emotion or complexity. In those moments, flexibility matters. The skill lies in knowing when to bend the structure and when to return to it. That balance is where genuine care lives.

A structured consultation is not robotic. It is a map through uncertainty.

16.2 Working with uncertainty

Some of the safest consultations do not end with a firm diagnosis. They end with clarity, reassurance and a plan.

In general practice, it is entirely appropriate for a consultation to conclude with a working diagnosis and clear safety-netting. A note that reads 'Likely viral illness. Safety-netting discussed. Review if worse' reflects thoughtful, proportionate care. It is not a failure. It is honest medicine.

Patients often respond well to openness about uncertainty when it is framed constructively. Saying *"let's keep an eye on this"* communicates vigilance rather than indecision, but it should always be followed by clear guidance on what to watch for. It reassures patients that you are engaged, cautious and prepared to adapt if circumstances change.

There are times when naming uncertainty explicitly builds trust. Saying *"I'm not completely sure what's happening yet, but we'll work it out together"* does not undermine authority. It humanises you and invites the patient into a shared process of monitoring and review.

Becoming comfortable with uncertainty helps you avoid unnecessary investigations and referrals. It allows you to pause when appropriate, to monitor safely, and to recognise when time itself is a diagnostic tool.

16.3 Managing time in the room

Ten minutes can be enough to reach a safe and effective outcome when the consultation is gently guided.

Curiosity matters. Open questions matter. Silence sometimes matters too. But allowing the consultation to drift without direction often increases stress for both doctor and patient. Midway summaries help anchor the conversation. Returning to "so *what I'm hearing is...*" recentres both of you and keeps focus on what matters most.

Managing multiple issues is one of the most common challenges. Patients frequently arrive with lists, some explicit and some implied. A respectful negotiation is essential. Saying *"you've mentioned a couple of things; which feels most important to focus on today, and could we arrange another appointment for the rest?"* protects safety while preserving rapport.

Gentle redirection can be done without shutting patients down. If detail becomes overwhelming, phrases such as *"let's come back to that at your review"* or *"would it be okay if we pause that and pick it up next time?"* keep the relationship intact.

Time management is a soft skill. It develops through repetition, reflection and small adjustments rather than through speed alone. The aim is not efficiency at all costs, but rhythm.

16.4 What about the list?

Your task list will never be finished, and that is not a personal failing. It is the nature of general practice.

Trying to solve everything in one consultation often creates more work later. Prioritising value over volume makes care safer and more sustainable. Ask yourself what carries risk today, what matters most to the patient today, and what genuinely needs action today.

Using the flow of your clinic helps. Short, straightforward consultations can be used to clear results or admin. More complex presentations deserve longer appointments or planned follow-ups. Saying *"let's book another appointment so I can give this the attention it deserves"* is a mark of professionalism, not inadequacy.

Learning your own pace matters. Notice how long you tend to take for history, examination, prescribing and documentation. Awareness allows you to flag early, adapt and reduce frustration.

If you need more time, booking a follow-up is not failure. It is care.

16.5 What I wish I had known

Your ten minutes with a patient is not about fixing everything. It is about connection, clarity and direction.

Most patients are not asking for a complete solution in one sitting. They want to feel heard, understood and safe. When you listen carefully, explain clearly and agree on next steps, ten minutes can be enough. Sometimes it can be more than enough.

Some of the most effective consultations end with an invitation rather than a conclusion. Saying *"I want to understand this better, so let's review it in two weeks"* demonstrates safety, curiosity and respect for complexity. That is medicine at its best.

Ten minutes is enough to listen, focus and make a plan.

Final thought

Learning to work in ten minutes is not about speed. It is about judgement. Over time, you will become more comfortable deciding what needs attention now and what can safely wait. That skill develops quietly, through practice and reflection, not through pressure.

When you use structure thoughtfully, accept uncertainty honestly, and set clear boundaries kindly, ten minutes becomes workable. Not perfect, but safe, humane and effective.

Reflective prompts:

- How do you use the opening minute of a consultation to establish focus and rapport?
- Think of a consultation where uncertainty felt uncomfortable. What helped you hold that space safely?
- How do you negotiate multiple problems without losing sight of the patient's main concern?
- When was the last time you booked a follow-up because time ran out, and how did the patient respond?
- What phrase helps you bring a consultation to a clear and compassionate close?

CHAPTER 17
The paperwork and the ePortfolio

"Yes, it's admin. But it's also your story. Tell it well."

The ePortfolio can easily feel like an unwelcome companion during GP training. It sits quietly in the background while you juggle clinics, exams, supervision and life outside work. When time is tight, it can feel like an added burden rather than a meaningful part of your development.

But the portfolio does not have to be something you endure. With the right mindset and habits, it can become a practical tool for reflection, self-awareness and growth. Used well, it becomes a record not just of what you have done, but of who you are becoming as a GP.

17.1 Making the ePortfolio work for you

Your ePortfolio is not an exam paper and it is not a diary. It is a professional narrative. You are not writing bullet points to satisfy a supervisor; you are documenting your development as a doctor in progress.

A simple structure helps. Many trainees find it useful to anchor reflections around three questions: what went well, what was difficult, and what you would do differently next time. This keeps entries focused, readable and genuinely reflective. Over time, these entries quietly map your journey. When you look back, the difference between how you wrote as an ST1 and how you reflect as an ST2 or ST3 becomes striking.

Write as if you are speaking to your future self. Include what you felt as well as what you thought. Anxiety around a challenging consultation, frustration with time pressure, or uncertainty about risk are all worth naming. Noticing emotional responses is not a weakness; it is evidence of insight and honesty. Reflection that acknowledges feeling is often where the most meaningful learning sits.

Avoid turning entries into long diary-style accounts. Length does not equal depth. A clear, structured reflection of 200 to 300 words is usually far more effective than a sprawling narrative that loses focus. Setting a rough target of around

150 words can help keep entries manageable while still capturing context, insight and next steps.

You're not writing for your supervisor. You're writing for your future self.

17.2 Understanding WPBAs

Workplace-based assessments can feel like boxes to tick when you are busy. In reality, they are mirrors. Used well, they reflect how you think, communicate and practise, and they highlight where you are progressing and where support might help.

Case-based discussions are about reasoning rather than outcomes. Supervisors are interested in why you chose a particular approach, how you weighed risk, and what alternatives you considered. Even a case that went smoothly can generate valuable discussion if you focus on your thinking rather than the result.

For COTs or SCA cases, choose variety rather than polish. A mix of presentations such as paediatrics, mental health, long-term conditions and complexity tells a more honest story than selecting only your strongest performances. Training is about breadth and learning, not about appearing flawless.

Mini-CEX and DOPS work best when they are frequent and low-pressure. Waiting for the perfect case often means missing useful learning opportunities. Routine consultations are excellent for practising communication, examination or prescribing, and they are usually easier for supervisors to observe.

Patient and staff feedback provide insight into your interpersonal style. Positive comments can be reassuring, but neutral or critical feedback is often where growth lies. Pay attention to where patients felt listened to and where clarity could have been improved.

Each WPBA contributes to a broader professional picture. Approaching them with intention, such as deciding what kind of feedback you want in a given week, makes them far more meaningful.

Perfect scores are overrated. Impactful learning isn't.

17.3 How to reflect without cringing

Reflection does not need drama to be valuable. It is not reserved for things that went wrong. At its best, it is a form of professional mindfulness, helping you notice nuance, reinforce strengths and anticipate challenges.

Simple prompts often work best. What surprised you in the consultation? What felt satisfying or aligned with your values? Where did you hesitate or pause? These questions shift reflection away from self-criticism and towards curiosity.

If something felt uncomfortable, explore why. It might relate to communication style, fear of missing something important, time pressure, or emotional resonance with the patient's story. Insight lies not in assigning blame, but in noticing patterns.

Many trainees find it helpful to write in the present tense. Saying that you felt unsettled when a patient asked about lifestyle, and that you noticed yourself rushing, keeps reflections grounded and honest. If writing about feelings feels awkward, remember that feelings are data. They show you where you care, where you may struggle, and where you are growing.

You don't need drama to learn, just curiosity.

17.4 Staying organised without burning out

The ePortfolio is not a one-off project. It is ongoing maintenance, and small habits make it manageable.

A weekly rhythm works better than sporadic bursts of effort. Setting aside a regular 30-minute slot, perhaps during a quieter lunch break or after work, helps maintain steady momentum without overwhelm. Keeping a simple note, whether on your phone or in a notebook, allows you to capture potential reflection ideas as they arise.

Each week, aim to convert one of those notes into a reflection, WPBA or feedback entry. This might be a challenging consultation, a piece of informal feedback or a learning point from teaching. Consistency matters more than volume. Two entries a week is excellent. One is still progress.

Use routine admin to your advantage. Mandatory teaching, learning logs and feedback from MSFs can all contribute content. Reviewing your entries at the end of each month can highlight gaps and help you plan future learning more intentionally.

Sharing draft bullet points with your supervisor before reviews can also help focus conversations. Letting them know what you are working on invites more meaningful discussion and guidance.

Doing a bit regularly beats burning out at year-end.

17.5 What I wish I had known

No one expects you to love the portfolio, but you may come to respect it once it becomes genuinely yours.

It is not a tick-box exercise. It is a record of growth. When you look back after a year, you will see moments where anxiety softened into confidence, where uncertainty became safer decision-making, and where difficult experiences led to insight.

If entries feel flat, add colour. Include brief quotes from patients, feedback from supervisors, or moments of personal realisation. Track small victories as well as challenges. The first time you asked for help and changed your plan. The first time you safely reassured and discharged someone. These moments matter.

Not every entry needs polish. Strong reflection is about depth, not literary flair. When stuck, sharing a draft with a peer who is slightly ahead in training can provide perspective and reassurance.

The portfolio is a mirror. It reflects what you notice, what you value, and how you are growing.

Final thought

The ePortfolio is not there to catch you out. It is there to slow you down just enough to notice who you are becoming.

In the rush of clinics, assessments and everyday demands, it is easy to move from one patient to the next without pausing to register the learning. The ePortfolio creates that pause. It asks you to step back and make sense of your decisions, your emotions and your growth. It invites you to see patterns rather than isolated moments.

Used reluctantly, it feels heavy. Used intentionally, it becomes something steadier: a quiet companion to your development. Long after individual cases are forgotten, what remains is how you learnt to think, how you learnt to ask for help, and how you learnt to carry responsibility.

The paperwork may feel administrative. The growth it captures is deeply professional and quietly transformative.

Reflective prompts:

- How does writing for your future self change the way you approach portfolio entries?
- Which type of WPBA do you find most meaningful, and what does that say about your learning style?
- What emotion has surprised you most in recent reflections, and what might it be pointing towards?
- What small routine could you adopt to keep your ePortfolio manageable?
- When you look back at early entries, what signs of your own development stand out?

CHAPTER 18

What no one tells you about working solo

"You're not alone – but it will feel like it sometimes."

At some point in your training, often sooner than you expect, you will open your clinic list and realise something has changed. There is no trainer in the next room. No familiar knock on the door. No quick, whispered question between patients.

Just you, a computer and a list of names waiting to be called.

This moment is a quiet rite of passage in general practice. It does not arrive with ceremony or warning. And for many trainees, it brings a sudden, unsettling awareness of responsibility.

18.1 The quiet weight of responsibility

Even when supervision is technically available, by phone, message or at the end of the session, the shift is real. You are the one making the decision. It is your name on the notes, your explanation the patient leaves with, your plan that carries forward.

That responsibility can feel heavier when no one else is physically present.

You may notice yourself sitting a little straighter, thinking a little longer and re-reading your notes before you press 'save'. These are not signs of anxiety; they are signs that you are stepping fully into the role.

Being on your own does not mean you are unsupported. But it does mean you will grow faster than you expected.

18.2 You will overthink (almost) everything

Did I miss something subtle? Was my safety-netting clear enough? Should I have escalated?

These questions often surface once the door closes and the patient has gone. They can loop quietly in your mind long after the clinic ends.

This kind of overthinking is common and, within limits, healthy. It reflects awareness, caution and care. But it can also be draining if left unchecked.

Build in space after solo sessions to decompress. Talk things through with a supervisor. Write down unresolved questions to revisit later. Learning does not stop when the clinic ends – it often begins there.

Reflection sharpens judgement; rumination dulls it. Learn to tell the difference.

18.3 You might miss the 'little questions'

One of the less obvious challenges of working solo is the loss of informal learning. The small, corridor-style questions that shape practice quietly over time:

- *"Would you have examined that?"*
- *"What would you code this under?"*
- *"Would you safety-net that differently?"*

These moments may seem minor, but they accumulate into confidence and clinical nuance.

When you work alone, those opportunities pause. Try to reclaim them later. Bring questions to your supervisor. Discuss cases in tutorial time. Ask about the decisions you almost made but didn't.

Much of GP training happens in these small, reflective spaces, not just in formal assessments.

18.4 Your confidence will feel wobbly

One consultation may feel smooth and satisfying. The next may leave you doubting everything you just did. This fluctuation can be unsettling, particularly when no one else has witnessed the encounter.

This is not failure. It is growth.

You are learning to trust your process, even when no one is watching. You are discovering how you think, how you tolerate uncertainty, and when you need to pause or escalate.

There is an important difference between being alone and being unsupported. One is temporary, but the other is optional, if you speak up.

18.5 You are allowed to pause

If possible, protect a short administrative or catch-up slot during solo sessions. Use it intentionally: to review notes, reflect, breathe or reset.

No clinician functions well at full cognitive and emotional speed for hours on end, particularly when the work involves risk, responsibility and human distress.

Taking a pause is not weakness. It is professionalism.

18.6 What I wish I had known

I wish I had known that feeling uneasy in solo clinics does not mean you are unsafe. Often, it means you are becoming more aware of the weight of decisions and learning to carry them thoughtfully.

Confidence in general practice does not arrive all at once. It builds quietly, case by case, decision by decision, especially in moments when you realise you managed something on your own, and did it well enough.

Final thought

Working solo is a strange blend of excitement and unease. It is where your GP identity begins to stretch, strengthen and take shape.

You do not need to be perfect. You need to be thoughtful, safe and willing to keep learning.

And remember: just because the door is closed does not mean help is far away. Sometimes it is only a phone call, or a message, away.

Reflective prompts:

- How did your first solo clinic feel, and what surprised you most about it?
- What internal voice tends to surface when you are working alone – supportive, critical, cautious?
- How do you balance speed and thoroughness when there is no one to ask mid-consultation?
- When you feel uncertain but cannot ask immediately, how do you flag or review those cases later?
- What single habit helps you feel more grounded during a solo session – note-making, brief pauses, breathing or structure?

CHAPTER 19
When you feel out of your depth

"It's not about knowing everything. It's about knowing when to stop, pause and ask."

There will be moments in GP training when your stomach drops. A patient may look more unwell than expected, mention a symptom that changes the whole picture, or reveal something that makes you realise you are no longer sure what you are dealing with. These moments are not simply clinical uncertainty, they are also about emotional safety, help-seeking, and learning the quiet discipline of not pretending.

Feeling out of your depth is not a sign that you do not belong. It is often a sign that you are paying attention. The goal is not to avoid these moments, but to recognise them early and respond in a way that protects both patient and clinician.

19.1 Recognising the feeling

Uncertainty is a clinical finding. Treat it with respect.

Sometimes the shift is subtle. You may notice a tightness in your chest, a brief loss of fluency, or the sense that your thoughts are circling the same question. You might find yourself thinking, "what do I do now?" or "have I missed something?". These internal cues are not a glitch. They are often your mind flagging uncertainty, risk, or a mismatch between the story and the conclusion you were about to reach.

In general practice, this internal signal matters. It is one of the earliest warnings that the consultation has changed direction. It may point to a red flag you have not yet explored, a differential that needs to be widened, or a decision that requires a second pair of eyes. It may also reflect emotional discomfort, such as a safeguarding concern, a boundary challenge, or a patient story that has landed in a way you did not expect. Either way, it deserves attention rather than dismissal.

When you notice that hesitation, ask yourself one simple question: What is this feeling trying to tell me? Even a brief pause, lasting only a few seconds, can be enough to regain clarity. Many mistakes in primary care are not caused by lack of knowledge. They arise when we push past uncertainty too quickly and treat the discomfort as something to suppress rather than something to investigate.

You are not a robot, and you are not meant to be. That inner voice can be a professional ally. If your instinct says pause, it is often your judgement asking for time to catch up with the pace of the consultation.

19.2 What to do in the moment

Pausing isn't hesitation. It's how you make space to think clearly.

When you feel out of your depth, the most useful first step is deceptively simple. Slow down, take a breath and sit back slightly. Allow your thinking to become deliberate rather than reactive. A brief pause can restore control in a consultation that is starting to feel uncertain.

It is entirely appropriate to say something like *"give me a moment to think that through"* or *"I want to get this right, so I'm going to check something quickly"*. These phrases do not undermine trust. They often increase it. Most patients do not expect instant certainty. What unsettles them is bluffing, abrupt reassurance, or a plan that feels rushed.

Once you have slowed the pace, anchor yourself with safety. Ask, "what am I worried about?", "what do I need to rule out today?". In many consultations, your job is to ensure you are not missing the urgent or serious possibilities before you settle on the most likely explanation. This is where basic red-flag thinking helps. Is this potentially life-threatening, rapidly progressive or time-critical? Are there signs of severe infection, acute neurological change, acute coronary syndrome, respiratory compromise or safeguarding risk? Have you checked observations when they matter, or assumed they are normal because the patient looks 'okay'?

If the consultation is complex, it is reasonable to acknowledge that openly. Practise a phrase you can use without apology: "*this is a bit more complex than I'd like to manage alone, so I'm going to discuss it with a colleague*". Said calmly, it signals responsibility rather than uncertainty. You are not asking for permission. You are explaining good practice.

If you still feel uneasy, do not carry it in silence. Step out if needed. Speak to your supervisor, duty doctor or on-call colleague. If you are working in an integrated team, involve the right professional. Safety in general practice is often built through conversations: the quick corridor check, the call between patients, the shared plan written clearly. Being safe is rarely a solo act.

19.3 Who to ask, and how

The strongest clinicians don't go it alone. They build networks of support.

Many trainees assume that asking for help always means asking the trainer. In reality, safe general practice is supported by the whole team, and the right person to ask depends on the question.

Practice nurses often hold deep, practical wisdom. They can guide you through wound care decisions, immunisation queries, chronic disease nuance, or what usually works for that community. Pharmacists are invaluable for interactions, formulary choices, side-effect profiles and safer prescribing. Reception and admin colleagues know local services, referral patterns and what is realistic in your area. Community teams can help you make sense of social context, follow-up capacity, and the hidden constraints shaping a patient's life. Senior GPs and clinical supervisors remain key, particularly for risk, diagnosis and decision-making, but they are not the only source of insight.

How you ask matters. Vague questions often invite vague reassurance. Aim for a brief statement, your working impression, and a clear question. For example: "*I have a patient with chest discomfort, a normal ECG, and symptoms that don't fit typical angina. My concern is whether I'm missing something time-critical. Could I run my thinking past you?*". This shows you have assessed, you have a concern, and you are seeking a specific steer.

When you receive useful advice, capture it. You do not need a lengthy portfolio entry every time. A short note on what you asked, what you learnt, and what you will do next builds clinical memory. Over time, these small learning loops become confidence. They also protect you from repeating the same uncertainty in future consultations.

If appropriate, close the loop. Let the person who advised you know what happened next. That follow-up strengthens relationships and deepens learning.

19.4 When it happens again

It's not about never being out of your depth. It's about knowing how to find the shore again.

This will happen again, and that is not a sign that you are regressing. Repetition is part of training. In fact, each time you pause, seek support and reflect, you are teaching your nervous system a new response. Early on, uncertainty can trigger racing thoughts and a strong urge to act quickly. Over time, you learn a different rhythm. You pause sooner. You ask sooner. You tolerate not knowing without panicking.

You may hope that the sinking feeling disappears completely. In most clinicians, it never does, and that can be a good thing. What changes is not whether you feel it, but how you respond. You begin to recognise that discomfort is not danger. You learn that you can rely on tools, checklists, colleagues and time. You build a personal process that turns fear into action.

There is value in sharing these experiences with peers and supervisors, not as confession, but as professional learning. Saying I felt out of my depth with this presentation, so I paused, checked the red flags, spoke to a colleague and adjusted the plan is not weakness. It is how safe clinicians think. It helps others feel less alone and builds a culture where uncertainty can be named and managed rather than hidden.

Celebrate progress, not perfection. The small changes matter. The moment you pause before prescribing. The moment you choose observation over reassurance. The moment you say, I'd like a second opinion on this. Those are professional milestones.

19.5 What I wish I had known

Confidence in general practice isn't certainty. It's knowing how to stay steady in the fog.

Early in training, I believed confidence meant being sure. With time, I learnt that general practice rarely offers complete certainty. What matters is steadiness. A calm approach to uncertainty, a reliable safety process, and the humility to involve others when needed. These are not signs of weakness. They are the foundations of safe primary care.

There is also an important distinction between not knowing the diagnosis and not being able to handle the consultation. The first is common and often honest. The second is usually the inner critic speaking too loudly. You may not always know what something is, but you can still manage it safely. You can ask the right questions, examine carefully, check observations, identify red flags, and make a plan that includes review and escalation when needed.

Medical school teaches you what to think. Hospital training teaches you what to do. General practice teaches you how to hold uncertainty while still being accountable. There is no shortcut to that skill, but it grows through repetition, reflection and support.

When you learn to steady yourself in uncertainty, you are practising courage. That is far more useful than perfection.

Final thought

Being out of your depth does not mean you are drowning. It often means you have reached deeper water, where your judgement is developing and your safety instincts are being tested. Each time you pause, ask and reflect, you are learning how to swim with steadiness and humility. You are not doing this alone. Help is part of the job, and learning to reach for it early is one of the most important clinical skills you will ever acquire.

Reflective prompts:

- Think of the last time you felt out of your depth. What was the first moment you noticed the shift, and what helped you steady yourself?
- Which part of uncertainty is hardest for you: the clinical risk, the emotional pressure, or the fear of being judged?
- Who do you turn to most often for advice, and what makes that person or role helpful?
- How do you record the learning from these consultations so it becomes usable next time?
- What phrase helps you pause in a consultation without sounding uncertain or defensive?

CHAPTER 20
Asking for help as a clinical skill

"Not knowing isn't the problem. Pretending you do is."

Every GP trainee, no matter how bright, diligent or capable, will need to ask for help, often frequently. Asking questions is not a transitional phase you grow out of; it is a professional habit you grow into. It underpins safe decision-making, reflective practice and long-term resilience.

Yet despite this, asking for help often carries an emotional charge. You may worry about appearing inexperienced, slowing others down, or revealing a gap you think should already be filled. These thoughts are rarely voiced, but they shape behaviour quietly and powerfully.

This chapter exists to name that discomfort, dismantle it, and replace it with something healthier and more sustainable.

20.1 Asking for help is professional

You are not expected to have all the answers. Not in your first week. Not in your first year. And, if we are honest, not even at the end of your career.

General practice is defined by uncertainty; symptoms evolve and context matters. Decisions are made with incomplete information. The safest clinicians are those who recognise early when uncertainty exceeds their comfort and pause to check their thinking.

Competence includes knowing your limits. It does not involve pretending those limits do not exist.

As a trainer and appraiser, I have seen that the most concerning doctors are not those who ask questions, but those who never do. Silence can sometimes be a sign not of confidence, but of fear.

20.2 Make it easier for yourself

One reason asking for help feels difficult is that the moment itself can feel exposed. Having a familiar phrase ready reduces the emotional load and turns help-seeking into a routine professional exchange. Examples that work well include:

- *"Can I just run something by you quickly?"*
- *"I'm comfortable with my plan, but I'd like to sense-check it – do you have a moment?"*
- *"I've got a patient with X. My thinking is Y. Is there anything you'd approach differently?"*

Notice the structure: you are not presenting confusion, but reasoning. You are showing that you have thought carefully and are inviting collaboration. This is how experienced clinicians speak to each other every day. You are not asking permission – you are practising medicine safely.

20.3 Choose your moment (but don't wait too long)

There is rarely a perfect moment to ask for help in a busy surgery; doors are closed, patients are waiting and everyone looks occupied.

But timing should never trump safety.

Most supervisors would far rather be interrupted early than be called later to untangle uncertainty that has already escalated. A brief check at minute three can prevent a cascade of doubt at minute thirty.

If your supervisor is mid-consultation:

- Jot a clear reminder to yourself and return at the next gap, or
- Say, "*Could I catch you between patients about a quick clinical question?*"

You are not inconveniencing someone – you are behaving as a responsible colleague.

20.4 It gets easier with practice

The first few times you ask for help, your heart rate may rise. You may rehearse the question in your head. You may apologise unnecessarily. But over time, something changes and you begin to recognise patterns:

- When uncertainty signals genuine risk
- When management needs confirmation rather than overhaul
- When reassurance, from a senior or yourself, is sufficient.

This process is how clinical judgement forms. It cannot be taught purely from books or guidelines. It emerges through repeated cycles of decision, reflection and dialogue.

Good clinicians do not know everything. They know when to pause, when to ask, and when to proceed.

20.5 Notice the response – not just the fear

The anticipation of asking is often worse than the reality. Pay attention to what actually happens when you do ask:

- You are listened to.
- Your thinking is respected.
- You leave with clarity, reassurance or a useful adjustment.

Each of these moments deposits quiet confidence. Over time, help-seeking stops feeling like exposure and starts feeling like professional connection.

It also models good behaviour. Trainees who ask thoughtful questions tend to create safer teams wherever they work later on.

20.6 What I wish I had known

I wish I had known earlier that asking for help does not diminish authority – it strengthens it. Supervisors are not looking for flawless performance; they are looking for honesty, curiosity and insight.

The doctors who struggle most are often those who carry doubt silently. Unshared uncertainty is far heavier than shared uncertainty.

Medicine was never meant to be practised alone.

Final thought

You are not here to impress. You are here to learn.

Help-seeking is not a weakness; it is a cornerstone of safe, resilient medical practice. The earlier you normalise it for yourself, the more likely you are to foster a culture of openness and safety for others.

So ask. Ask early. Ask thoughtfully.

You are not just seeking support – you are learning how to practise medicine well.

Reflective prompts:

- What is one question you hesitated to ask recently, and what stopped you?
- How do you usually feel after asking for help – relieved, embarrassed, reassured or validated?
- What internal language could you use to make help-seeking feel safer and more routine?
- Think of a time someone asked you for help. How did you respond, and what did that teach you about collaboration?
- What would asking for help 'with confidence' sound like in your own voice?

CHAPTER 21
Managing imposter syndrome

"You're not here by accident. You earned this, and you belong."

At some point during GP training, often quietly and without warning, a familiar doubt may surface. You might find yourself questioning whether you truly deserve your place, whether you know enough, or whether at some stage someone will realise you are not as capable as they think. These thoughts can be unsettling, particularly when they arrive in the middle of busy clinics or after a consultation that did not go as smoothly as you hoped.

This experience has a name, and it is far more common than most trainees realise. Imposter syndrome is not a sign of incompetence or failure. More often, it reflects responsibility, insight and a genuine desire to practise well. This chapter is not about eliminating self-doubt entirely, which is neither realistic nor necessary. It is about learning to recognise imposter syndrome for what it is, understanding how it operates, and developing ways to work alongside it without allowing it to undermine your confidence or your enjoyment of general practice.

21.1 Recognising it for what it is

Imposter syndrome is not about a lack of ability. It is about the gap between how competent you feel and how competent you actually are. In medicine, and particularly in general practice, that gap can feel wide because the work is complex, relational and often uncertain.

Paradoxically, the more reflective and conscientious you are, the louder the internal critic can become. Doctors who think carefully about their decisions are often more aware of what they do not know. That awareness can easily be misinterpreted as inadequacy.

Learning to name the feeling is an important first step. Simply acknowledging it to yourself, perhaps by thinking "I'm having an imposter day today", can reduce its hold. Once named, it becomes something you can observe rather than something that silently shapes your behaviour.

Confidence is rarely the starting point. It is usually the outcome of repeatedly showing up, practising safely, and continuing even when certainty is absent.

21.2 You are not alone, even when it feels that way

One of the most difficult aspects of imposter syndrome is the sense of isolation it creates. It can feel as though everyone else is coping effortlessly while you are struggling internally. In reality, this impression is almost always misleading.

Trainees at every stage experience self-doubt. Newly qualified GPs feel it when they first practise independently. Senior clinicians encounter it when faced with unfamiliar situations, complex risk or change. The difference is not that doubt disappears with experience, but that it becomes more recognisable and less frightening.

If you ever find yourself thinking that you are the only one who feels this way, it is worth remembering that self-doubt tends to be loudest in private. Others may simply be better practised at carrying it quietly.

Feeling uncertain does not mean you are failing. It means you are engaging seriously with a role that carries real responsibility.

21.3 Stop waiting to feel ready

Many trainees fall into the trap of believing that one day they will suddenly feel like a GP, and that until then they are somehow pretending. This moment rarely arrives in a clear or dramatic way.

General practice does not wait for you to feel fully prepared. It asks you to work thoughtfully, to seek support when needed, and to keep learning as you go. You do not need to feel confident all the time to provide safe and compassionate care. What matters far more is curiosity, humility and an openness to feedback.

You are not required to feel invincible or certain. You are required to be honest about uncertainty and willing to address it.

Becoming a GP is a gradual process. It unfolds through everyday consultations rather than through a single moment of confidence.

21.4 Gathering your evidence

Imposter syndrome is selective in what it remembers. It clings to hesitation and uncertainty while quietly discarding evidence of competence and growth. One way to counter this is to consciously collect evidence that tells a fuller story.

This evidence is often modest rather than dramatic. It might be a patient who returned because they trusted you, or a consultation you handled safely despite feeling unsure at the time. It may be clear documentation written under pressure, or feedback from a trainer that recognised your thoughtfulness.

Some trainees find it helpful to keep a simple record of these moments, sometimes called a confidence file. This can be a notebook, a document or a few lines written at the end of a challenging day. Returning to these reminders on more difficult days can help rebalance perspective.

Feelings are powerful, but they are not always reliable narrators of your progress.

21.5 Redefining what success looks like

If your internal definition of success is perfection, you are likely to feel like a fraud regardless of how well you practise. Medicine does not allow for perfection, and general practice in particular involves working with uncertainty, time pressure and incomplete information.

A more realistic and sustainable definition of good practice asks different questions. Did you recognise what you did not know? Did you act safely and honestly? Did you seek advice when it mattered? Did you treat the patient in front of you with care and respect?

These are the foundations of good general practice. They are far more meaningful than an illusion of flawless performance.

Perfection is not the goal. Safe, kind and reflective practice is.

21.6 Talking about it

Imposter syndrome thrives in silence. It loses much of its power when spoken aloud.

Simple statements such as *"I felt really out of my depth in that consultation"* or *"today was a bit of an imposter day"* often invite unexpected responses. Colleagues frequently reply with recognition rather than judgement, sometimes saying that they feel like that too.

These exchanges do not undermine professionalism. They strengthen it by creating a culture where uncertainty can be shared and managed safely. Medicine can be isolating work, particularly in general practice where much of the day is spent behind a closed door. Speaking openly about doubt reminds us that we are not carrying this responsibility alone.

Final thought

Imposter syndrome rarely disappears completely, and it does not need to. Over time, its voice usually softens as experience accumulates, evidence is gathered, and uncertainty becomes more familiar. You may not feel like a GP every single day, but general practice is not sustained by feelings alone. It is sustained by actions, by showing up consistently, thinking carefully, and caring for patients even when confidence wavers.

You are not here by accident. You earned your place. With time and experience, you will come to recognise that you belong, even on the days when it does not feel that way.

Reflective prompts:

- When did you last question your place in GP training, and what seemed to trigger that feeling?
- What would you say to a colleague who expressed the same doubts you sometimes carry?
- Can you identify three recent moments that demonstrate your development as a GP?
- How do you speak to yourself after a mistake or a difficult consultation, and would you use the same words with a friend?
- What thought or phrase might help you ground yourself on days when self-doubt feels particularly strong?

CHAPTER 22
Feedback, failure and finding your way

"If you've never felt like you failed, you probably weren't learning anything new."

Feedback in GP training arrives in many forms. Some of it is formal and expected, such as workplace-based assessments and supervisor reports. Some arrives unexpectedly as a brief comment after clinic, a critical email, a patient complaint, or a look from a colleague that stays with you longer than it should. Some feedback will feel fair, timely and helpful. Some will feel clumsy, unbalanced or difficult to hear.

At some point, something will go wrong. It may not be dramatic, but it may be enough to shake your confidence. You might miss a nuance in the history, underestimate risk, choose words that land poorly, or later realise you could have handled a consultation differently. This chapter is about how to receive feedback with maturity, how to learn from error without becoming defined by it, and how to develop a grounded sense of what being a good GP means to you.

22.1 When feedback stings

Feedback isn't always fair, but it can still be fertile ground.

It is a common experience to finish a clinic feeling you have done reasonably well, only to be thrown off course by a comment that catches you unprepared. Sometimes it is a supervisor pointing out something you missed. Sometimes it is an email that feels sharp in tone. Sometimes it is a complaint that makes you replay a consultation in your mind long after you have gone home. Even small feedback can feel disproportionate when you are already tired, stretched and trying hard.

If your first response is defensiveness or hurt, that is normal. Your professional identity is still forming. When it is challenged, even gently, the instinct to protect yourself is human. The skill is not in pretending you are unaffected. The skill is in avoiding a reflex response that closes down learning.

In the moment, it helps to pause and take a breath. Thank the person, even briefly, and give yourself time to reflect before responding in depth. A simple sentence such as *"thank you, I'll think about that"* buys you space without diminishing your professionalism. It allows you to step away from the immediate sting and return with a clearer mind.

With time and distance, look for the kernel of truth. Even poorly delivered feedback may contain something useful. Ask yourself what the person might be seeing that you have not yet recognised. Consider whether there is a pattern emerging, or whether a particular consultation style is repeatedly being misunderstood. You do not have to accept every piece of feedback as correct, and you are allowed to disagree with tone or context. But it is worth examining feedback with curiosity before you decide it has nothing to offer.

In training, some of the most painful feedback turns out to be the feedback you needed most, even if it arrived in an imperfect form.

22.2 When you get something wrong

At some point during GP training, you will get something wrong. It might be a missed diagnosis, an underestimation of risk, a consultation that did not go well, or a plan that looks less sound in hindsight. It might involve a patient complaint or an uncomfortable debrief with a supervisor. These experiences are not rare, and they are not evidence that you should not be doing this job. They are part of the reality of working in a complex system with limited time and incomplete information.

There is no such thing as a flawless GP. Those who appear effortlessly competent have usually built that steadiness over years, often carrying their own stories of missed opportunities, hindsight learning, and difficult moments that shaped their practice. Mistakes are not the opposite of competence. They are often part of how competence is formed.

What matters most is what you do next. It takes integrity to acknowledge what happened, to be honest about your role in it, and to engage actively with learning rather than avoidance. Owning a mistake is not the same as drowning in shame; shame paralyses, but integrity clarifies.

There are times when an apology is needed, and a simple, sincere acknowledgement can go a long way. What matters is that it is grounded, proportionate and patient-centred. At the same time, resist the urge to spiral into catastrophising. One error does not erase the good work you have done, and it does not define your future practice.

If something has gone wrong, reflect in a structured way. Ask what happened, why it happened, and what you will do differently next time. Consider system factors such as workload, time pressure, interruptions and unclear pathways, as well as personal factors such as fatigue, stress and emotional resonance with the case. A clear reflection is not just a portfolio task. It is a way of turning pain into learning, and learning into safer practice.

You can own a mistake without being consumed by it.

22.3 Finding your own shape as a GP

You don't need to be the fastest or the slickest. You need to be yourself, safely.

One of the quieter challenges in GP training is the gradual realisation that there is no single 'right' way to be a GP. Early on, it is easy to compare yourself to trainers, to peers, or to the polished clinicians you have shadowed. You may admire someone's speed, their diagnostic sharpness, their warm humour or their unflappable calm. You may also notice styles that feel less aligned with your values. This is all part of the process.

General practice contains a wide range of consulting styles. Some doctors are quick and instinctive. Others are methodical and careful. Some connect through warmth and conversation. Others through clarity and calm. You will try different approaches, keep what fits, and discard what feels unnatural. Over time, you will develop a style that is recognisably yours.

It helps to identify who you admire and why. Pay attention not only to their knowledge, but to how they hold the room. Notice how they speak when they are uncertain, how they negotiate time, how they handle difficult emotion, and how they safety-net without scaring patients. These qualities are not simply 'personality'; they are skills, many of which can be learnt and adapted without becoming a copy of someone else.

You do not need to be perfect, but you do need to be present. Patients rarely remember the exact phrasing of your plan, but they remember whether you seemed rushed, dismissive, attentive or kind. A GP who is slightly slower but thoughtful and safe can be outstanding. A GP who consults quietly but listens deeply can be transformative. The aim is not to become a superhero clinician. It is to become a reliable, reflective doctor who keeps learning.

General practice needs doctors who bring themselves to the consultation, not just the guideline.

22.4 What I wish I had known

You can make mistakes and still be a good doctor.

No one really prepares you for how personal feedback can feel when you are still becoming a doctor in the community. A single critical comment can stick more firmly than a dozen thank-yous. Even when you have done your best, you may carry the sense that you have let someone down. That burden is common, and it can be heavy.

With experience, you learn that good doctors are not those who never get knocked. They are those who keep returning to the work with humility and steadiness. Some days you will feel bruised by feedback or misunderstood by a system that is under pressure. You may question your place. You may question whether you are cut out for this. Those moments do not mean you are failing. They mean you are doing something demanding, and you care about doing it well.

Let go of the myth of the flawless GP. The clinicians you respect most have often been shaped by hard moments. Confidence is rarely constant. Growth is rarely linear. What matters is your willingness to reflect, to repair where needed, and to keep improving without losing your compassion for yourself.

You do not need to be fearless. You need to be steady. You need to remain open to learning. You need to keep showing up, particularly after the difficult days.

Final thought

Feedback will shape you, but it does not get to define you. You will receive comments that are insightful, and others that are clumsy or unfair. You will have days where you surprise yourself in a good way, and days where you walk home replaying every sentence. The direction you take is shaped by what you choose to do with these experiences.

If you can pause rather than react, learn rather than spiral, and reflect without cruelty, you will grow into a GP who is not only clinically capable, but emotionally durable. That is the kind of doctor patients trust, and the kind of colleague teams rely on. Most importantly, it is the kind of doctor you can sustain being.

Reflective prompts:

- What piece of feedback has stayed with you, and why do you think it mattered?
- When something does not go well, what is your inner voice like, and is it kind or harsh?
- What does being a 'good GP' mean to you now, and how has that definition shifted during training?
- Think of a mistake or near-miss that changed your practice for the better. What did you learn, and what will you repeat next time?
- Which GPs do you admire most, and what qualities would you like to develop in your own way?

CHAPTER 23
Support, safety and looking after yourself

"You can't pour from an empty cup, but you don't have to wait until it's dry to refill it."

GP training is demanding in ways that are not always visible from the outside. It is intellectually stretching, emotionally absorbing, and often carried out under time pressure with a steady stream of human need in front of you. Burnout is real, isolation is common, and many trainees keep going without ever stopping to ask themselves a simple question: "am I actually okay?".

This chapter is about noticing strain early, knowing where to turn, and understanding that self-care is not indulgent, but is professional integrity. A GP who is supported, rested and emotionally steady will listen better, think more clearly and practise for longer. Looking after yourself is not separate from patient care. It is one of the things that makes patient care safer.

23.1 Recognising the signs

Burnout doesn't look like failure. It looks like pushing through.

Many trainees do not realise they are struggling until they are already deep into overwhelm. That is partly because medicine rewards endurance. You learn early to keep going, to show up, to cope. The difficulty is that burnout rarely announces itself as collapse. More often it arrives as a quiet shift in your baseline.

One early sign is feeling drained before the day has even begun. Most people feel some apprehension before clinic, but if dread becomes frequent, if you wake with heaviness and fatigue that does not lift, it is worth taking seriously. It does not mean you are weak. It usually means you are running low on reserves.

Irritability, cynicism or emotional numbness are also common warning signs. You might find yourself snapping at small things, feeling impatient with colleagues, or noticing a hard edge creeping into your internal dialogue. Sometimes it is not irritability but detachment. You feel less moved by stories that would normally matter to you. You still care, but you feel disconnected from your own purpose. These changes can be subtle, and that is exactly why they are easy to miss.

Avoidance is another clue. You might delay finishing notes, put off supervision, or find yourself procrastinating before clinic. These behaviours are rarely laziness. They are often the mind trying to protect itself from more demand. Unfortunately, avoidance tends to create a second wave of stress, because unfinished tasks breed guilt and further overwhelm.

Sleep disturbance, anxiety and unexpected tearfulness can also be part of the picture. You may feel restless at night, wake early with a racing mind, or feel emotionally fragile in a way that surprises you. These are not signs of incompetence. They are signals that your system is under strain and asking for care.

These signs matter because burnout affects clinical practice. When you are depleted, your listening becomes thinner, your patience shorter, and your decision-making more vulnerable to error. Recognising the early signs is not simply kindness to yourself. It is part of your duty of care.

If anything in this list feels uncomfortably familiar, start with a small step. Name it honestly, even if only to yourself. Then decide what support would make the next week safer and more manageable.

23.2 Where to find support

"You don't have to reach crisis point to ask for help."

One of the hardest things in training is not the clinical work. It is the moment you recognise you are struggling and still hesitate to speak. Medical culture often prizes independence and resilience, and trainees can feel that admitting difficulty will be judged as weakness. In reality, thriving in general practice does not happen in isolation. It happens in conversation.

Your clinical supervisor is often the most appropriate starting point, particularly if the relationship feels safe and respectful. You do not need a polished explanation. A simple sentence such as *"I don't think I'm coping as well as I'd like right now"* can open the door to practical changes, such as adjusted workload, closer supervision, or help prioritising what matters. Good supervisors are not only assessing your learning. They are also part of the safety-net around you.

If the issue feels too personal, too complex, or simply hard to discuss within the practice, your training programme can help. Training programme directors and scheme wellbeing leads exist for exactly this reason. They will not be shocked. They have seen these pressures before, and many have lived them themselves. Early support can prevent a difficult period from becoming a crisis.

Peers are often the most powerful source of normalisation. Other trainees are in the same landscape, even if they appear to be coping better. A quiet message to a trusted colleague can bring relief and perspective. In many areas there are Balint groups, trainee peer groups, or facilitated reflective spaces, and it is worth engaging with them if they are available.

There are also external, confidential options that many doctors find helpful. Practitioner Health is widely used by clinicians who need confidential mental health support. The BMA offers counselling and peer support for members. Your own GP matters too. Doctors need doctors, and registering with a GP and using that care when needed is part of being a safe professional.

Support is not reserved for breakdown. It is also for early signs, maintenance and prevention. You are allowed to ask for help simply because you do not feel like yourself and want to address it early.

23.3 Self-care is not optional

Rest is not a luxury. It is your foundation.

Self-care can sound like a soft concept until you have experienced what exhaustion does to your thinking and your compassion. In reality, it is just physiology and psychology. When you are under-fuelled and under-rested, your tolerance shrinks and your clinical reasoning becomes more brittle.

Start with basics because basics are not basic when you are busy. Eat in a way that sustains you through the day rather than simply patching hunger. Drink water, because dehydration quickly affects mood and concentration, and it is surprisingly common in clinic-heavy days. Move your body, even briefly. A short walk between sessions, a stretch, or a few minutes outside can reset attention more than people expect. Protect sleep where you can. Regular sleep is not a lifestyle goal. It is part of cognitive safety.

Make space for something that has nothing to do with medicine. This is not a reward you earn when everything is done. It is part of how you stay human. Whether it is music, sport, photography, cooking, reading, faith, community or being outdoors, it matters because it reminds you that you are more than your workload.

Protect your time off. If your day off becomes a day of catching up on admin, it stops doing its job. Training is demanding, but rest is not optional. A boundary is only a boundary if it is kept, even when guilt tries to negotiate.

Small moments also count. A deep breath before the next patient. A brief pause after a difficult conversation. A short walk at lunch rather than eating at the desk. These micro-resets do not solve everything, but they reduce the sense of relentless pressure and remind you that you have agency.

When you reframe self-care as professional integrity, it becomes easier to prioritise. Looking after yourself supports safer prescribing, more patient-centred consultations, and better teamwork. It also models good practice for colleagues and future trainees. You do not have to be self-sacrificing to be admirable, but you do have to be sustainable.

23.4 What I wish I had known

You're not a machine. You're a human being doing a human job.

In training, it is easy to treat rest as something you must earn. You begin to believe you can pause only when you have finished everything, and because everything is never finished, you keep going until you are running on fumes. I wish I had understood earlier that you do not have to wait for a crisis to deserve support.

Compassion fatigue is real. If you feel yourself hardening, disconnecting, or dreading the next consultation, those are not moral failures. They are signs that you have been giving a lot, often quietly, and you need replenishment. The answer is not to become tougher, it is to become more self-aware.

I also wish I had known how normal it is for doctors to struggle in silence. There is no medal for doing that. Asking for help is not a flaw. It is a strength and a safety skill. A short conversation, early, can change the direction of a difficult month.

Finally, I wish I had protected my life outside medicine more deliberately. General practice is a career that can take up as much of you as you will give it. Keeping parts of yourself intact is not selfish. It is protective. You are not only a GP. You are also a person, and the person deserves care.

Burnout is not inevitable. There are habits, boundaries and supports that make a difference. It is easier to refill when the cup is half-empty than when you are scraping the bottom.

Final thought

Looking after yourself is not the opposite of being a good GP. It is part of the job description. Your wellbeing shapes your attention, your empathy, your judgement and your capacity to keep turning up with steadiness. If you can notice strain early, reach for support without shame, and protect a life outside work, you will not only survive training. You will become the kind of GP who can do this work with humanity for the long term.

Reflective prompts:

- What are your early warning signs that you are becoming stretched, physically or emotionally?
- Which person or group currently helps you feel safe and understood, and how could you strengthen that connection?
- What is one non-medical activity that restores you, and what would it take to protect time for it each week?
- When have you pushed through for the sake of being 'professional', and what did it cost you?
- What boundary do you most want to improve, and how might that boundary make you a safer clinician?

PART 4

LOOKING AHEAD

"GP training is a phase. General practice is a career. What you build now will shape what follows."

CHAPTER 24
Finding your GP identity

"You're not 'just a GP'. You're a specialist in complexity, continuity and compassion."

At some point, often quietly, the language around you changes. You are no longer described as 'in training'. You are introduced simply as the GP. Patients stop asking how much of your training you still have to do, and start asking when you are next in. Colleagues begin to treat your opinion as settled rather than provisional.

And yet, if you are honest, you may not feel fully formed.

This chapter is about that space. The space between qualification and confidence, between competence and identity. It is about recognising that becoming a GP is not something that finishes with CCT. It is something that continues, shaped by experience, values, boundaries and choice.

Finding your GP identity is not about deciding everything now. It is about noticing who you already are in the consulting room and giving yourself permission to grow into that, rather than moulding yourself to fit an imagined ideal.

24.1 GPs don't all look the same

One of the most liberating realisations in general practice is that there is no single correct way to be a GP.

Some doctors are drawn to dermatology, enjoying the clarity of visual diagnosis and pattern recognition. Others thrive in safeguarding work, navigating complexity with patience and moral clarity. Some find deep satisfaction in mental health, long-term conditions or end-of-life care. Others discover energy in urgent care, leadership, teaching, research or quality improvement.

None of these paths is more 'proper' than another. What matters is that your practice is safe, reflective and sustainable.

Early in your career, it is easy to assume that confidence looks like speed, decisiveness or encyclopaedic knowledge. With time, you begin to notice that patients often value something quieter. Being listened to. Being remembered. Being taken seriously. Being met with calm rather than certainty.

You bring something unique to the consulting room. Your background, your temperament, your life experience, your way of speaking and listening all shape the care you give. Owning that does not mean ignoring standards. It means practising within them in a way that is honest and humane.

24.2 Discovering what you enjoy

Your clinical interests often reveal themselves gradually.

Pay attention to the consultations that energise you rather than drain you. Notice which cases you keep thinking about, not because they worry you, but because they intrigue you. Observe the feedback you receive from patients and colleagues. Sometimes they see your strengths before you do.

You may find that you explain things clearly, and patients leave reassured. You may notice that colleagues come to you with questions about a particular area. These are not accidents. They are early signals.

Exploration does not require commitment. Short courses, taster sessions, extended roles, or focused CPD can help you test interests without locking yourself into a path too early. Curiosity is enough at this stage.

Equally, it is important to notice what consistently depletes you. Disliking a particular type of work does not make you inadequate. It makes you human. Knowing this early allows you to shape a career that plays to your strengths rather than constantly compensating for your weaknesses.

24.3 Beyond the consulting room

For many GPs, identity eventually extends beyond clinical sessions alone.

Some find meaning in education and supporting trainees and students through the same uncertainties they once faced. Others contribute through leadership, service development or quality improvement. Some write, research, advocate or innovate. These roles can add richness and variety to a career, but they also require balance.

Portfolio careers are often spoken about as aspirational, but they are not a solution to dissatisfaction on their own. Adding roles without clarity can increase pressure rather than relieve it. The question is not how many roles you can hold, but whether they align with your values and capacity.

You do not need to decide any of this now. Staying open is enough. A career in general practice is long, and it is allowed to evolve. Many fulfilling roles emerge years after qualification, shaped by timing, opportunity and personal circumstance.

24.4 Boundaries are part of your identity

One of the least discussed aspects of GP identity is boundary setting.

The ability to say no to extra sessions, committees, or roles that do not fit you is not a failure of commitment. It is an act of self-knowledge. A week that sustains you will always serve patients better than one that quietly erodes you.

Your GP identity should support your life, not consume it. This includes how many sessions you work, how you structure your week, and how you protect time outside medicine. Boundaries are not rigid rules. They are living agreements between your work and your wellbeing, and they will change over time.

Learning to honour them early is one of the most important skills you will develop.

24.5 What I wish I had known

I wish I had known that it was acceptable to grow into my GP identity slowly.

For a long time, I thought identity was something you achieved, a settled sense of who you were once you had enough experience. In reality, it is something you practise. It lives in how you speak to patients, how you handle uncertainty, how you respond to pressure, and how you treat yourself after difficult days.

Your identity is not defined solely by what you do. It is shaped by how you do it, what you value, and the energy you bring into each room. Start there and the rest will follow.

Final thought

Being a GP is not about fitting a mould. It is about shaping a career that fits you, your values, and the life you want to lead. General practice is broad enough to hold many identities. Yours does not need to look like anyone else's to be valid.

You are not 'just a GP'. You are becoming a particular kind of GP, and that distinction matters.

Reflective prompts:

- Which types of consultations leave you feeling most engaged, and why?
- What strengths do patients or colleagues most often reflect back to you?
- What parts of GP work do you find consistently draining, and what might that be telling you?
- How comfortable are you with letting your career evolve rather than deciding everything early?
- What boundaries would help your GP identity support your life more sustainably?

CHAPTER 25

The road to CCT

"This isn't the end of the road. It's the end of the on-ramp."

ST3 often feels like a year lived in between. You are more independent, more capable and more trusted than ever before, yet you are still 'in training'. You lead clinics, make complex decisions, and hold risk with greater confidence, but the portfolio continues, the assessments loom, and the finish line feels both close and strangely distant.

This chapter is about making sense of that final stretch. It is not a checklist for passing. It is a guide to navigating the clinical, administrative and emotional work of transitioning from trainee to independent GP, while staying grounded and kind to yourself along the way.

25.1 What the final year really brings

By ST3, the tone of your working day has changed. Clinics are fuller and patients more complex. You may be covering duty doctor sessions, supervising others informally, or managing uncertainty with less immediate oversight. Supervision becomes lighter not because you are unsupported, but because you are trusted.

This shift can feel affirming and unsettling at the same time. Many trainees describe an 'almost there' feeling. You are tired, capable and quietly counting down. There can be pride in how far you have come, alongside impatience to be done and anxiety about what comes next.

It helps to remember that ST3 is not about proving yourself from scratch. It is about trusting the judgement you have already built. You are consolidating patterns of thinking, decision-making and communication that will carry you forward into independent practice.

ST3 isn't just about proving yourself. It's about trusting yourself.

25.2 Navigating the final assessments

The final assessments can easily dominate the emotional landscape of ST3. If you are preparing for the SCA, the pressure can feel disproportionate, especially when layered on top of full clinical work.

Preparation works best when it starts early and stays steady. Knowing the format well in advance allows you to practise without panic. Choosing cases that reflect everyday general practice is far more helpful than chasing rare or dramatic presentations. Examiners are looking for safe, structured thinking, clear communication and appropriate endings, not perfection.

Aim to demonstrate how you manage common problems well, how you recognise complexity, and how you safety-net clearly. Use peer groups, mock sessions, and local teaching where available. Feedback at this stage is not a judgement of your worth. It is fine-tuning.

It is also worth naming the emotional load. These assessments sit at the end of years of effort. Feeling nervous does not mean you are unprepared. It means this matters to you.

25.3 Finishing the portfolio without losing yourself

By ST3, the portfolio can feel relentless. Even confident trainees can feel overwhelmed by what still needs to be uploaded, mapped or signed off. The key is visibility and organisation rather than intensity.

Take time early in the year to review what remains. Use a simple checklist or planner so that nothing sits vaguely in the background creating anxiety. Spread the work out. Last-minute panic rarely produces good reflection.

As you write, focus less on volume and more on insight. Your supervisor is not looking for evidence that you have done everything perfectly. They are looking for evidence that you think clearly, learn from experience and practise safely. Showing how your reasoning has evolved is far more powerful than trying to impress.

Keep regular contact with your supervisor, not just for sign-off, but for perspective. These conversations often become more reflective at this stage, shifting from "what's missing?" to "how are you feeling about what comes next?"

25.4 ARCP and the moment of CCT

The ARCP is often misunderstood. It is not another exam to fear. It is a structured review of your journey, bringing together evidence of competence, reflection and progression. Attention to detail matters here. Make sure documents are uploaded, clearly named and correctly mapped. Administrative clarity reduces unnecessary stress.

CCT itself can feel strangely quiet when it arrives. There is often relief, pride and a sense of disbelief that this long chapter is closing. It is important to acknowledge it because this is not just a certificate. It represents years of learning, uncertainty, resilience and growth.

Celebrate it in a way that feels right to you. You have earned that moment.

25.5 What I wish I had known

I wish I had understood that you do not finish training as a 'complete' GP. You finish as a safe, thoughtful clinician who is ready to keep learning independently. That is the point.

Flying solo can feel daunting at first, but it is not the same as being alone. Support does not disappear with CCT. It simply changes shape. Colleagues, mentors, peer networks and your own judgement remain part of the picture.

The most important transition in ST3 is not administrative. It is internal. You begin to trust that you can hold uncertainty, ask for help when needed, and continue to grow without a training label attached.

That confidence arrives quietly, often after you have already earned it.

Final thought

The road to CCT is not a sprint to an endpoint. It is a merging lane, preparing you to join the wider flow of general practice with confidence and care. When you reach it, you may still feel moments of doubt, excitement and humility. That is not a problem. It is a sign that you understand the responsibility you are stepping into.

You are not just finishing training. You are stepping forward as the GP you have been becoming all along.

Reflective prompts:

- What aspects of ST3 have helped you trust your judgement more?
- Which parts of the final year feel most stressful, and what support has helped?
- How has your approach to uncertainty changed since ST1?
- What kind of support will you seek once formal training ends?
- How do you want to mark the moment of CCT in a way that feels meaningful to you?

CHAPTER 26

What happens after training?

"CCT is not the finish line. It is your licence to shape your future."

Many doctors expect qualification to feel triumphant. Instead, what often follows is something quieter and more confusing. The exams are done, the portfolio is closed, and the structure that has carried you for years suddenly falls away. In its place sits freedom, choice and an unsettling question: What now?

This chapter is about preparing for that transition. It explores the emotional dip that can follow CCT, the realities of choosing your first post-training role, and how to approach your early months as a fully qualified GP with clarity rather than urgency.

26.1 The post-CCT dip

For many newly qualified GPs, the weeks after CCT bring a mixture of relief and disorientation. The pressure that sustained you through training eases, and with it the adrenaline that kept everything moving. Without warning, the rota disappears, supervision becomes optional, and there is no longer a portfolio demanding regular reflection.

This loss of structure can feel destabilising. Some describe a sense of anticlimax, others a return of imposter syndrome. You may find yourself asking whether you are really ready, despite years of evidence to the contrary. These feelings are common, and they do not mean you have made a mistake or reached the wrong destination.

It helps to create your own rhythm early. Simple routines around work, rest and reflection can provide continuity while you adjust. Remember that confidence after CCT rarely arrives overnight. More often, it creeps in quietly, noticed only in hindsight.

CCT doesn't make you feel different. One day, you will simply realise that you are.

26.2 First jobs and early choices

One of the most immediate questions after training is what form your work should take. Locum, salaried and partnership roles each offer different opportunities and challenges, and none is inherently superior.

Locum work can provide flexibility, exposure to different practices, and higher hourly pay. It can also feel isolating, with variable support and limited continuity. Salaried roles often offer stability, mentorship and predictable income, although sometimes with less autonomy. Partnership brings influence, leadership and long-term investment, alongside business responsibility and shared risk.

Early on, many GPs benefit from trying a mix. Short-term roles can help you understand what suits your temperament, values and energy. There is no requirement to decide your entire career in the first year after CCT. Choosing curiosity over commitment often leads to better decisions later.

26.3 Choosing the right practice

When considering a practice, look beyond geography and job title. Team culture matters. Support matters. Ask about workload, admin processes, supervision, clinical meetings, breaks, and home visit expectations. These details shape your day far more than a job description ever will.

If possible, visit the practice. Pay attention to how people speak to one another, how problems are discussed, and whether there is space for questions. Trust your instincts. A supportive environment in your first post-training role can make the difference between steady growth and early burnout.

26.4 Transitioning roles with humility

After CCT, you are no longer a trainee, but you are still learning. That truth matters. Accepting support does not undermine your status. It protects your practice.

Be honest about what you know and what you are still developing. Ask questions. Seek mentorship. Reflect as you always have. Mistakes will still happen, because medicine remains complex. What changes is your relationship with those mistakes. You are no longer being assessed, but you are still responsible for learning from experience.

Staying reflective after training is one of the strongest predictors of long-term professional satisfaction.

26.5 What I wish I had known

I wish I had known how normal it is for the first year after CCT to feel unsettled. I expected clarity and confidence. What I found instead was choice, and with it uncertainty. Over time, I learnt that no first job defines your entire career. Paths change. Interests evolve. What feels right now may not feel right in five years, and that is not failure.

The goal after training is not to feel settled immediately. It is to stay safe, connected and open to growth. If you can do that, the rest unfolds in its own time.

Final thought

After training, you do not suddenly become a 'real' GP. You already are one. The difference is that you now have the freedom to decide what kind of GP you want to be, and how you want your work to fit into your life.

Take that freedom seriously, but not fearfully. You have earned the right to shape what comes next.

Reflective prompts:

- What emotions surfaced for you after finishing training, and which surprised you most?
- What kind of support do you want in your first post-CCT role?
- How do you balance flexibility with the need for belonging and continuity?
- What would a good first year look like for you, beyond job titles?
- How will you continue reflective practice once the portfolio has gone?

CHAPTER 27

A career that grows with you

"You're not choosing a job. You're beginning a relationship with a profession that can change as you do."

One of the quiet strengths of general practice is its capacity to evolve. Unlike many medical careers that narrow with time, general practice can widen, soften, deepen or shift direction as your life changes. It can accommodate growth, retreat, reinvention and return.

This chapter is not about career planning in the traditional sense. It is about taking a long view. It invites you to step away from the pressure to design a perfect future and instead build a career that remains sustainable, flexible and meaningful over decades, not just years.

27.1 A career, not a job

Early in your working life, it is easy to think in terms of roles. Locum or salaried. Partner or portfolio. Urban or rural. These choices matter, but they are not the whole story.

General practice is better understood as a living ecosystem. You can move within it, step back from it, or lean into it at different stages of your life. You can pause clinical work for family, health or personal reasons. You can retrain, refocus, slow down or scale up. Very few decisions in general practice are irreversible.

Many GPs look back and realise that the career they imagined at qualification bears little resemblance to the one they now value most. That is not drift. It is evolution.

Longevity in medicine is not about endurance. It is about adaptation.

27.2 Building sustainability

Burnout does not automatically mean you are in the wrong profession. Often it means the rhythm of your work no longer matches the rhythm of your life.

Sustainability begins with honesty. Notice what drains you and what restores you. Pay attention to how many sessions you work, how your week is structured, and how much emotional labour your role demands. These factors matter as much as job title or income.

A sustainable career makes space for the rest of your life. Relationships, health, creativity, rest and interests outside medicine are not distractions from your work. They are what allow you to keep doing it well.

You do not need to be productive all the time to be valuable. There will be seasons of intensity and seasons of consolidation. Learning to respect those cycles is one of the most important professional skills you will develop.

27.3 Making the career your own

General practice offers extraordinary scope for shaping a career that reflects who you are.

Some doctors develop clinical special interests in areas such as dermatology, musculoskeletal medicine, mental health or women's health. Others find meaning in education, teaching medical students, trainees or the wider healthcare workforce. Leadership roles within practices, primary care networks or local systems can offer influence and challenge beyond the consulting room. Some GPs are drawn to innovation, digital health, health equity or quality improvement work.

You do not need to pursue all of these, and you do not need to decide now. Interests often emerge through experience rather than planning. What matters is staying open and responsive to what energises you rather than what you think you should want.

A career that feels personal is more likely to be one you can sustain.

27.4 What I wish I had known

I wish I had known earlier that there is no rush to arrive at a final version of yourself as a GP.

Early on, I felt pressure to define my niche, to commit to a direction, to demonstrate ambition. With time, I learnt that listening to my own energy, instincts and limits mattered far more. Careers are shaped as much by life events as by professional aspirations, and both deserve respect.

Your needs will change. Your priorities will shift. What fulfils you now may not fulfil you later, and something unexpected may take its place. That is not instability. It is responsiveness.

The freedom to evolve is one of the greatest gifts of general practice. Use it.

Final thought

A GP career is not something you complete. It is something you live alongside the rest of your life.

If you allow it to grow with you, to bend when needed, and to reflect who you are becoming rather than who you once were, it can remain a source of purpose and meaning for many years.

You do not need to map the entire road ahead. You only need to stay attentive to yourself as you travel it.

Reflective prompts:

- How do you imagine your ideal working week might look five or ten years from now?
- What aspects of general practice currently give you the most energy?
- Where do you notice strain, and what might that be telling you about pace or boundaries?
- Which interests would you like to explore gently, without committing too early?
- What would a sustainable, fulfilling career mean to you personally?

CHAPTER 28

In case no one told you

"You've made it this far, not because it was easy, but because you kept showing up. That matters more than you know."

Dear reader,

By the time you reach these pages, you have already done more than you probably give yourself credit for. You have sat through induction sessions that blurred together, navigated consultations that stayed with you long after the door closed, absorbed feedback that stung, and written reflections when you would rather have slept. You have comforted anxious parents, supported patients at their most vulnerable, and made careful decisions under pressure when there was no obvious right answer.

You have grown. Not just in clinical skill, but in presence. You have learnt how to listen without rushing, how to pause when something does not feel right, how to ask for help, how to hold uncertainty, and how to care even when you felt tired to the bone. These are not small things. They are the quiet foundations of good general practice.

This chapter is not here to tell you what to do next. It is here to remind you of what you already carry.

This may feel like the end of a book, but it is really a moment of transition. Your role may be changing, your responsibilities may be widening, and your confidence may still feel uneven. That is normal. Titles shift more quickly than identities do. What matters most is not that you feel ready all the time, but that you continue to practise with integrity, curiosity and care.

In case no one told you, you are allowed to still have questions. You are allowed to feel uncertain some days and capable on others. You are allowed to take your time becoming the GP you will eventually recognise as your own. Confidence in this profession does not arrive all at once. It settles gradually, through repetition, reflection, and the steady accumulation of lived experience.

You do not need to know everything. You never will. What your patients need is not perfection, but safety, kindness and attentiveness. They need someone who is willing to listen properly, to explain honestly, and to act thoughtfully. They need a doctor who remains human in a system that can sometimes feel anything but.

You are not a machine. Your energy is not infinite. Protecting it is not selfish; it is professional. A depleted doctor cannot listen as well, think as clearly, or care as generously. Looking after yourself is part of the work, not something separate from it.

The GP you are becoming does not need to resemble anyone else. There is no single correct way to practise. Your temperament, your values, your pace, and your way of being with patients are not weaknesses to be ironed out. They are strengths to understand and refine. Difference is not a flaw in general practice; it is one of its greatest assets.

Trust your instincts. When something feels off, pause. When you are unsure, ask. When you feel overwhelmed, speak up. None of these actions diminishes you. They are signs of judgement, maturity and care.

Before you close this book, take a moment to consider one final question.

What do you want the patients you care for to feel after they have seen you, spoken with you, or sat with you in the consulting room?

Whatever your answer is, let it guide your choices. Let it shape how you practise, how you set boundaries, and how you define success for yourself. A career built around that intention will be one that remains meaningful, even when the work is hard.

You have already shown that you can keep going. More than that, you have shown that you can keep caring.

You have got this. And general practice is genuinely fortunate to have you.

With warmth and belief,

Hussain Shakir

"Let the end of this book mark the beginning of a successful and fulfilling career in primary care."